# MS TALENT

Volume 1: A collection of short stories, poetry and memoirs

Edited by John Lake and Rachel Evans.

Published by Jasmine Cottage Publishing, England.

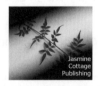

**MS TALENT** (First Edition)

**ISBN: 978-0-9557393-0-9**

First published in Great Britain by
Jasmine Cottage Publishing 2007

**www.mstalent.org**

A catalogue record for this book is available
from the British Library.

Published by: Jasmine Cottage Publishing, Gravel Hill, Gerrards Cross SL9 0NU.

Printed and bound in Great Britain by: CPI Antony Rowe Limited, Bumper's Farm, Chippenham, Wiltshire SN14 6LH. All CPI Antony Rowe's papers are Forest Stewardship Council approved.

# Introduction

The inspiration for this volume came from its contributors, all of whom have some connection with multiple sclerosis (MS). MS is the most common neurological disease affecting young people in the UK.

Publishing, printing, postage and packaging costs for the first edition have been met by private individuals – which means the whole of the donation for a first edition copy will go to bona fide charities dealing with MS in the UK, see page 184. If this is a later edition or reprint that you're reading, there may be slightly different arrangements, but the principle's the same.

Please be sure to tell your friends how brilliant it is so that they get their own copy. And meantime get saving for MS Talent Volume 2.

Thank you for your donation – it's made a difference. If someone has given you this book as a gift, please pass on our gratitude for their donation when you say your own "thank you".

Health warning: this book contains articles expressing opinions which we hope you will find interesting. The publisher, the editors and the MS charities benefiting from donations made for this book do not endorse these comments. We recommend that you seek professional medical advice relating to your own personal circumstances before commencing any therapy or treatment, whether mainstream or alternative.

# Dedicated

This volume is dedicated to all people with multiple sclerosis, and their families, friends and colleagues who support them in their everyday lives.

Special mention has to go to Barry Slade for coming up with so many ideas, our virtual friends Celia Fallon and Jennie Albinson for their help with reading and checking under pressure, Chalfont Photographic Services for their unstinting assistance and expertise and a host of other people who sat on the book's editorial panel and gave their time and valued opinions.

And a big thank you must also go to everyone else who so generously and patiently donated their time, money and of course their stories, poetry and personal accounts – including those we couldn't fit in – to make this volume a success.

Finally, this dedication wouldn't be complete without mentioning the long-suffering families of all the talented authors who submitted their work. Thank you all.

# Contents

**A selection of short stories**                    **9**

Justicia                                            11

Seahorses                                           13

A bridge called Sam                                 16

The hotel                                           21

Silvery threads                                     26

The shopping list                                   27

Crossroads                                          29

I don't feel like dancing                           30

Balancing act                                       37

A tale of two                                       42

Easter break                                        46

Taxi driver                                         48

On the mountain                                     50

Grandmother, cider and tales                        51

Mummy the fairy                                     54

The nearest W.C.                                    57

Better to live than dream...                        58

An exercise routine                                 64

Curve ball                                          65

I see Dot                                           71

**A selection of poetry**                           **73**

Wild country lane                                   75

As dreams go by                                     76

Poets corner                                        79

Bird of paradise                                    79

Shadow                                              80

Memo to self                                        80

Tour de England                                     81

Where are you?                                      81

A summer sonnet                                     82

M.S.                                           82
The old red lady                               83
Earth, sea and sky                             84
Feral youth                                    86
Aliases                                        87
Preacher/poacher                               87
Tidal strand                                   88
Storm dance                                    89
Flying lessons                                 91
Uninvited visitor......                        92
Swansea bay tide                               93
Carpe diem                                     93
9/11 – the orphans                             94
Where do you go?                               94
My cuckoo clock is broken                      95
Manifesting sunshine                           96
Only one square metre                          97
The dolphin poem                               98
Swept away (Tsunami 2004)                      99
I am that I am                                 100
Why should I feel half a woman?                101
If only for a moment                           101
For Callum                                     102
Meanings                                       103
Artist                                         104
Princess                                       105
Me!                                            106
The ballad of Znorbare                         107
**A selection of memoirs**                     **111**
In search of Paddington                        113
The Mystic Ferret's tale                       115
The dancer                                     116
The fence painting incident                    118

The PWDD AGM                          119
Another lazy Sunday afternoon         120
The ultimate Alpine challenge         123
And I haven't even got it             127
Combat techniques                     130
Emotional freedom technique           131
Help!                                 136
Some days                             140
Guilt                                 142
Can you jump tandem?                  144
A positive diagnosis                  148
Third eye                             152
Relapse and remission                 155
You had to be there                   161
In praise of Spanish healthcare       165
Passage to England                    169
My trip to Ottawa                     174
See, listen, remember                 180
About MS                              183
About the MS Society                  184
About the MS Trust                    186
About the MSRC                        188
About the Kent MS Therapy Centre      190

# A selection of short stories

# JUSTICIA

## By Krax the Mighty (2005)

Mama won't let me take off my hat. It's big and blue and the edges flop down in front of my eyes so all I can see is ground and blue. I push it back up a little bit as I walk next to her, but Mama tells me off and pushes it back down. I have to put my head right back to see her face, and her eyes are big and wide above her veil. She keeps looking back behind us too.

I'm a little frightened. I don't know where we are and Mama is making us rush down lots of dirty alleys. And it's all kinds of dirt, some like I've never seen before. The newspaper looks the same, but the dirt is wet like sludge around some of the big bins, round the corners mostly. Sometimes it comes up over the sides of our sandals and gets stuck under our feet, and we have to stop and rub our feet on the newspaper when it gets too annoying.

It's cold too, which I don't like. It's really hot outside of where the buildings are all close together, but in the gaps that we're in it's dark and chilly. I can't rub my arms because Mama is holding one of my hands, and I don't want one warm arm and one cold one. I think here it's like a fridge when the door is shut, or when the light's broken. I tell Mama that, and she nods at me and pulls on my T-shirt. She pinches my skin a bit but then rubs my neck to say she's sorry.

There's a sort of crossroad in the alley and Mama stops us right by the corner. She makes me stay behind her as she looks around the corner. She's still got my hand in hers but she's squeezing it too hard. I whine a bit and try to get my fingers out of hers, but she holds me tight and gives me a little jerk to tell me to be quiet. I put my fist by my nose and rub my hand by my mouth to help me.

Mama pulls me across the crossroad and I look down one of the alleys as we go. I can see the soldiers at the end marching. I think they're on parade. There are lots of people watching them, and I don't think they can see us all the way down here. I don't think they should see us, because Mama is trying to hide us in the alleys. I think we're somewhere we're not supposed to be, like at home when I go into the kitchen before dinner. If Mama wasn't pulling me so much I think I'd like this. It's like an adventure.

We're getting close now, Mama tells me, real close. There's a long alley now and it's all filled up with bins and things. I'm smaller than it all and I'm scared something will fall on me. I move into Mama's side so she can look after me, and I watch my feet so I don't have to look at any of it.

There's suddenly a big crashing noise and Mama pulls us into the wall between two bins. I'm really scared now and I can feel my heart in my chest. Mama holds me really tight and she has a hand around my mouth to make sure I'm quiet. I don't mind it much because she's done it before. I stay really still and try not to slip even though she's making me stand on stuff. There's another crash and then a rattle, and then this really big cat comes around the bin. It's skinny and sort of fluffy but bits of it are all stuck together. It looks at us and then goes back to wherever it lives. I hope it lives somewhere nice even though it scared us.

Mama lets go of me and I hurry to get off the stuff I'm standing on because I'm scared I'll fall over. She rubs her chest a little bit and looks around the alley. I wait in the middle in the little path that runs right past everything. After a little while she gets up and takes my hand again. We start walking again and I keep looking round for more cats so we don't have to be scared again.

I don't know we're there until Mama says we are, and I pretend to look happy even though it looks the same. There's some red stuff on the wall next to us, handprints and splotches, and there are old tins of red paint and big stacks of newspaper lying around. I can't read what's on the wall but Mama looks really happy about it. 'Justicia' is written the biggest and right up on the top, with all the handprints under it.

Mama lets go of my hand to go to the old paint and colours up her hand really red. I hold the sides of my hat by my ears so the front goes up and watch her. She makes a handprint on the wall with all the others, pressing it down lots of time to make sure it's really clear. Then she picks up some of the newspaper and rubs it all off, putting the painted newspaper in the big bin.

Mama doesn't seem so scared any more, and she picks me up and puts me on her hip. Holding me tight, she looks at the wall for a long time and smiles a bit. I watch the wall too, but I don't know why. Soon she puts me down and pulls my hat right down by my eyes again. Then she holds my hand again and starts taking us back down the alley. I put my hand on my hat to make sure it doesn't move and look around at the wall. Soon there are too many bins in the way to see it and I look back where we're going. Mama walks a bit slower now that we're going home.

# SEAHORSES

## By Krax the Mighty (2006)

Tominaga-cho, Gion, came to life in the early afternoon, before the purple of dusk seeped into the horizon behind the mountains and whilst the ground was still warm from the midday sun. Outside the ochaya, the subtle and electric voice of the shamisen lilted to the river, coaxed from its three taut strings by the deft fingers of the geisha. It puddled with the murmurs and delighted laughs of the people on the bridge, the children throwing chilled seahorses to the river dragon below. His scales were puckered and fringed, like an old slipper, and wafted as he twisted and coiled in the water. When the paper cones were empty, they threw them into the river and watched the dragon sink them with a stream of bubbles from a curled nostril, before sucking them into his teeth.

Inside the ochaya, the tatami were hot underfoot, and Otonashi shifted her feet minutely beneath her, sat on her heels and feeling the warmth seep up through her kimono. The shamisen had fallen still and quiet as the teahouse's honoured guest made a request to the musician geisha. He was poured a new cup of sake as he spoke.

Otonashi remained in the posture the last dance had left her in, her back held straight by the thick obi and her hands resting on her thighs, palms hovering over the silk. Her painted face was still, the subdued frown having threatened to crease and line the white coat of her skin as she read their lips. She knew the dance Daichi had asked to see, and she slipped a hand behind her to collect the fan tucked at the edge of the thick tatami mat.

Peripherally, she saw Makoto take up the shamisen and begin to pluck, singing low and quivering notes to accompany it. The faint gold ripples reached Otonashi quickly, pressing like a weak wind into her kimono and telling her skin the rhythm. She rose in one smooth motion, the round edge of the kimono splayed out like a platform, the stitched pattern falling straight. Her heavy sleeves slipped back past her wrists, her left hand hidden and the fan sliding open in her right.

The dance was at once elegant and effortless but equally controlled and challenging. Otonashi's thighs ached as she remained bent at the knee, turning her body back and forth with the flipping fan. Her eyes remained perfectly glazed, fixed ahead as she tipped and rocked her head, the sound ripples coming faster as the song progressed. Her free hand touched the air as if she were rippling the river outside, drawing eddies and furls in the golden arcs.

The river dragon purred against the reeds as his scales were stroked, the music dull and thudding to him but the dance light and caressing. There were no more seahorses plopping into the water, and he wondered if the children were going back to the seller's cart for more. After a few moments he decided that they were not, but he did not swim on upstream immediately. He waited for the dancing geisha to finish, and for the ghostly touches to end.

Afterwards, Daichi paid the ochaya mistress the geishas' flower money and, with a short bow to all three women, stepped out into the street. The ground did not hold the warmth as well as the tatami mats had, despite being in the sun, and Daichi was quietly glad his lacquered sandals lifted him away from the chill.

Walking up the steep steps that took him to the top of the bridge, he followed the gazes and pointing hands of the people to the river dragon. The dragon was running his claws through the listless water weeds, twining the fronds through his toes to pull them taut before snapping them free. Daichi watched the weeds flutter downstream until the wind-chimes of the ochaya played. The mistress had knocked them with her hand as a means of drawing the rickshaw man's attention.

Otonashi stepped into her wooden sandals easily, Makoto only touching the silk at her elbow when she too was ready to go. The mistress bowed lower than they and cast an eye over their obi to check the fans were with them. The shamisen was scuttled to the rickshaw in the small hands of a maid, the girl bowing clumsily before running back inside.

Their exquisite umbrellas shielded them from the sun, and Daichi watched the two women step up to and sit back in the rickshaw. The driver lifted the wooden forks and pulled straight into a jog. They disappeared quickly into the tightly knitted houses, leaving the riverside in seconds.

Looking back into the water, he saw that the river dragon had also departed. No doubt he was seeking another bridge with more children to throw chilled seahorses to him.

**About the author**
*Krax the Mighty is a transgressive writer living in Cheltenham and has her sights set on a Creative Writing PhD, with intentions to live and die in a university. She aims to begin lecturing in the next few years, and is currently writing her first novel. She can be contacted at krax.sintax@gmail.com.*

# A BRIDGE CALLED SAM

## By George Church (2006)

And underneath the bridge
there lived a terrible, ugly, one-eyed troll.
Nobody was allowed to cross the bridge
without the troll's permission
and nobody ever got permission.

Fable: The Three Billy Goats Gruff

If I were to fall, for sure, I would be killed. I imagined it. Falling one hundred feet and smashing onto the towpath below, baked hard by the mid-summer sun, maybe shattering my skull on the rounded blue bricks that edged the canal. My broken body rolling into the malevolent liquid and sinking to join the other dead animals suspended in the thick soup, leaving just a few pale balloons and the occasional bit of crap tipping the oily iridescent surface. To me the black canal, gleaming with thin rainbow ribbons of petroleum, seemed bottomless.

Five feet above my head is the road. Each time a vehicle passes over the vibration sends a shower of debris cascading down. Protecting my eyes I stare down at my scuffed shoes until the dust settles. I am perched high above the disused industrial canal, balancing precariously within the cast iron structure that supports the bridge. Fearfully I believe I can't move another step and that now I'm really stuck.

The girders are spaced closer together at this point and the headroom is greatly reduced, forcing me to stoop awkwardly and making my back ache. I'm near the centre of the bridge where the valley plunges to its deepest level, the ominous surface of the canal glinting and beckoning far below.

I've picked a tortuous path through the skeleton structure to reach this scary location. The start of the climb was difficult; stepping from the steeply sloping grass bank up to a narrow horizontal ledge built into the brick abutment.

With my back to the wall, my arms outstretched with palms flattened on the brickwork searching for a non-existent grip, I move out along the narrow stone projection, the ground quickly falling away. The ledge turns ninety degrees and passes under the road verge to meet the first of the iron struts. The struts criss-cross to form an unintentional and therefore dangerous trellis walkway stretching the length of the bridge. I climb inside the metal lattice and thread my way carefully across, some of the struts are so thin that I rock perilously on the instep of my shoes, and finally arrive at my present frightening position.

Now my feet refuse to let me move forward and, even more terrifying for a little kid, I'm unable to retrace my earlier steps and return to safe land. If I ever get out of this, I promise I will never be scared again. I lean forward against the vertical support I'm clutching and rest my hot cheek against it. Clinging closely to the strut I can smell the dust of past years, the rain unable to wash the grime away because of the umbrella effect of the bridge above. The pungent smell of the grey peeling oil paint and the metallic tang of cast iron invades my nose and adds to my feeling of dread.

I blink my eyes quickly and I force back the tears that are welling. I grip the support tightly and wish I had ignored the nagging impulse which has driven me to cross underneath the bridge. Bloody Hell!

Although in a state of terrified paralysis my thoughts, at least, escape and drift far away.

~ ~ ~ ~ ~

I'm called Tommy by all the people that really know me, except when I'm a nuisance to my Mom and then it becomes a snapped Thomas. Another friend of mine Robert is known as Bobby. He is a year older than me and everyone says Bobby is big for his age. He's crossed the bridge before, using the hard way I mean. He was the first to call the bridge Sam but whenever I ask why he simply replies you'll find out, maybe.

He lives only a few doors away (in fact all my friends are neighbour's kids) so I heard of his bad accident very quickly. He hadn't fallen from the bridge but he had been trying to cross Sam the hard way. He'd failed to get across this time and when he was rushing home to clean up for his dinner a car knocked him down. Eyewitnesses said that Bobby skidded thirty feet on his back right down the High Street.

He broke both of his legs and ruined his genuine leather bomber jacket, just bought for him by his father. Bobby's Mom had died giving birth to his sister Pauline and his Dad tried to compensate by buying both of them lots of really good stuff. This doesn't seem to help a lot and Bobby has become very quiet, in fact sometimes he seems invisible. We're good friends and poor old Bobby says he's never tried to cross Sam again, except by the normal way.

Bobby was with me at the time of the fight. We were sitting on a stone step during the morning break at school when the fight started, as usual, out of nothing. The quadrangle was packed with kids fooling around and my feet had been trodden on a couple of times. The next time this happened I shoved the kid away and instantly we were into a real fight. By magic (or so it always seemed when a fight started) we were surrounded by every kid in the school and we tried to punch it out inside a tiny jostling ring, the remaining kids outside the circle were trying like crazy to elbow in. A Master stopped the mayhem and I finished covered in bruises and with a bloody nose (most of this damage had been inflicted by the frantic spectators).

By the next day at school I had more or less forgotten the fight and then the classroom door opened and in walked my opponent of yesterday. I was summoned to the front of the class and asked by the Master if I wished to continue the fight, wearing boxing gloves, in the gym at the end of lessons. The other kid looked a lot bigger than I remembered and my stomach began to churn badly. It's one thing to have a scrap in the heat of the moment but to have a cold choice like this thrust on you in front of your classmates was quite different. Bloody Hell! I couldn't back down and so I gulped and forced myself to say yes all right. The Master then repeated the question to the other kid who, just barely audible, incredibly whispered no sir I don't.

I could have yelled with absolute relief but I just eyeballed the kid as if to suggest that yeah, he'd made the right decision and avoided being beaten up. It remains one of my finer moments.

~ ~ ~ ~ ~

Beneath the bridge my cheek hurts where it presses against the gritty support and with the pain my thoughts return to my current dilemma. I stretch my neck tenderly and rub my face against a dirty out-stretched arm, my hand still tightly clutching the beam. I realize bleakly that I must overcome my terror and face the next obstacle ahead; the formidable narrow midpoint of the bridge. I risk a glance downwards and my eyes sweep through the yellow and green valley. The dark canal bisects the grass-covered slopes like an open cut. The surface is millpond still and reflects an image of the late afternoon sun. It resembles the gleaming red eye of a watchful black snake. Small white clouds drift over the valley floor and as a few particles flicker up closer to the bridge I realize with astonishment the pale mist is composed of large white summer butterflies. At this moment I would give anything to have their gift of flight.

I peer apprehensively forward. The manoeuvre that is necessary to continue the crossing looks impossible. It involves leaving the diminishing framework, which provides a few meagre hand and footholds, in order to climb onto a large diameter metal pipe. There is clearly no way to hold the featureless pipe other than by gripping hard with my legs, like riding a horse bareback.

I prepare myself and inhale a few deep breaths. I wriggle nervously into position astride the big pipe and I sit as centrally as possible, my feet reaching down each side to the widest part of the cylinder. I begin to shuffle along, first extending my splayed hands forward and then, supporting my weight on my arms, I slide my now ragged behind along the pipe. If I lose my balance I will plunge into the valley, down to where the terrible black abyss is waiting for me. I have to bend my neck to avoid bumping my head on the underside of the road; my hair brushes and collects fragments of loose detritus. My legs scrape against the rusty metal cylinder and the inside of my knees become smeared with a mixture of blood and dust. The sun is falling quickly in the sky and the underside of the bridge is now permeated with warm sunlight. As I reach the exact centre of the bridge, illuminated by the ruby sun, I see an embossed inscription cast into the midpoint iron beam. The words read GALTON BRIDGE and underneath in smaller letters Samuel Galton 1829. I squint at the beam with watery dust-filled eyes and sigh deeply yeah okay Bobby. I get it now!

Lying forward almost flat on the pipe, I squeeze under the inscribed beam and continue over the bridge. My confidence increases as I pass each successive beam and then unbelievably I am side-stepping gingerly along the far side stone ledge. I jump down onto the wonderful grassy earth on the other side of the bridge. A few white butterflies remain scattered in the cooling air and close to the ground the fragile creatures look small and vulnerable. In the past I've caught them easily with a thrown jacket and not many survived this rough treatment. Recalling how the butterflies sailed so freely beneath the bridge, I determine never to trap another one. I'm hot, tired and unbelievably filthy. I remember wearily I should have been home by now. My knees are skinned raw and mottled with greyish red patches but as I walk homewards, with the appearance of a diminutive scarecrow, I feel a sense of exhilaration. I've crossed old Sam the hard way and if nobody was there to witness my crossing, well so what?

Happily I wipe my damp forehead with my sleeve, spreading more grimy streaks across my face and I smile to myself with growing delight at my achievement. With the final moments of the disappearing sun, I turn briskly into the road where I live and then hear the distant and rather desperate voice of Mom calling Thomas.

Although I'm very late I dare not tell Mom where I've been. I know that if I do, for sure, I will be killed. Bloody Hell!

Then he lowered his horns, galloped along the bridge
and butted the ugly troll.
Up, up, up went the troll into the air...
then down, down, down into the rushing river below.
He disappeared below the swirling waters,
and was gone.

~ ~ ~ ~ ~

Author's note: The real name of the bridge called Sam is Galton
Bridge and it crosses the Galton Valley, which is now a protected
and important area of West Midlands industrial heritage. It was cast
at the Horseley Iron Works in Tipton. The wide Birmingham Canal
lies seventy-five feet below the centre of the bridge. Samuel Galton
was a Board Director of the Birmingham Canal Company. Thomas
Telford designed the fabulous bridge and it measures one hundred
and fifty feet across the span. At the time of its construction in
1829 it was the longest single span bridge in the world.

As a little kid I crossed over Galton Bridge, on my own, the hard
way.

# THE HOTEL

## By "D. Jones"

Dear Maid

Please do not leave any more of those little bars of soap in
my bathroom, since I have brought my own bath-sized
Imperial Leather.

Please remove the six unopened little bars from the shelf
under the medicine chest and another three in the shower
soap dish. They are in my way.

Thank you.

D. Jones

*Dear Room 814*

*I am not your regular maid. She will be back tomorrow, Thursday, from her day off.*

*I took the 3 hotel soaps out of the shower soap dish as you requested.*

*The 6 bars on your shelf I took out of your way and put on top of your Kleenex dispenser in case you should change your mind.*

*This leaves only the 3 bars I left today which my instructions from the management are to leave 3 soaps daily. I hope this is satisfactory.*

*Sophie, Relief Maid*


Dear Maid

I hope you are my regular maid.

Apparently Sophie did not tell you about my note to her concerning the little bars of soap. When I got back to my room this evening I found you had added 3 little Camay's to the shelf under my medicine cabinet.

I am going to be here in the hotel for two weeks and have brought my own bath-size Imperial Leather so I won't need those 6 little Camay's which are on the shelf. They are in my way when shaving, brushing teeth, etc. Please remove them.

D. Jones


*Dear Mr. Jones*

*My day off was last Wed. so the relief maid left 3 hotel soaps which we are instructed by the management.*

*I took the 6 soaps which were in your way on the shelf and put them in the soap dish where your Imperial Leather was. I put the Imperial Leather in the medicine cabinet for your convenience.*

*I didn't remove the 3 complimentary soaps which are always placed inside the medicine cabinet for all new check-ins and which you did not object to when you checked in last Monday.*

*Please let me know if I can of further assistance.*

*Joyce (your regular maid)*


*Dear Mr. Jones*

*The assistant manager, Mr. Baldwin, informed me this morning that you called him yesterday evening and said you were unhappy with your maid service. I have assigned a new girl to your room.*

*I hope you will accept my apologies for any past inconvenience. If you have any future complaints please contact me on extension 15488 between 8 a.m. and 5 p.m. so I can give it my personal attention.*

*Thank you.*

*Deborah Houghton*
*Housekeeper*


Dear Ms Houghton

It is impossible to contact you by phone since I leave the hotel for business at 7.30 a.m. and don't get back before 6 p.m. That's the reason I called Mr. Baldwin last night.

You were already off duty. I only asked Mr. Baldwin if he could do anything about those little bars of soap. The new maid you assigned me must have thought I was a new check-in today, since she left another 3 bars of hotel soap in my medicine cabinet along with her regular delivery of 3 bars on the bath-room shelf.

In just 5 days here I have accumulated 24 little bars of soap. Why are you doing this to me?

D. Jones

*Dear Mr. Jones*

*Your maid, Sophie, has been instructed to stop delivering soap to your room and remove the extra soaps. If I can be of further assistance, please call extension 15488 between 8 a.m. and 5 p.m. Thank you.*

*Deborah Houghton* ,
*Housekeeper*


Dear Mr. Baldwin

My bath-size Imperial Leather is missing! Every bar of soap was taken from my room including my own bath-size Imperial Leather. I came in late last night and had to call the bellhop to bring me 4 little bars of Pears.

D. Jones


*Dear Mr. Jones*

*I have informed our housekeeper, Deborah Houghton, of your soap problem. I cannot understand why there was no soap in your room, since our maids are instructed to leave 3 bars of soap each time they service a room.*

*The situation will be rectified immediately. Please accept my apologies for the inconvenience.*

*John Baldwin*
*Assistant Manager*


Dear Ms. Houghton

Who the heck left 54 little bars of Camay in my room? I came in last night and found 54 little bars of soap. I don't want 54 little bars of Camay. I want my one bar of bath-size Imperial Leather!

Do you realize I have 54 bars of soap in here?! All I want is my bath size Imperial Leather. Please give me back my bath-size Imperial Leather.

D. Jones

*Dear Mr. Jones*

*You complained of too much soap in your room so I had them removed. Then you complained to Mr. Baldwin that all your soap was missing so I personally returned them. The 24 which had been taken and the 3 you are supposed to receive daily.*

*I don't know anything about the 4 bars of Pears. Obviously your maid, Sophie, did not know I had returned your soaps so she also brought 24 plus the 3 daily. I don't know where you got the idea this hotel issues bath-size Imperial Leather.*

*I was able to locate some bath-size Palmolive which I left in your room.*

*Deborah Houghton*
*Housekeeper*


Dear Ms. Houghton

Just a short note to bring you up-to-date on my latest soap inventory. As of today I possess:

On shelf under medicine cabinet - 18 Camay in 4 stacks of 4 and 1 stack of 2.

On Kleenex dispenser - 11 Camay in 2 stacks of 4 and 1 stack of 3.

On bedroom dresser - 1 stack of 3 Pears, 1 stack of 4 hotel-size Palmolive, and 8 Camay in 2 stacks of 4.

Inside medicine cabinet - 14 Camay in 3 stacks of 4 and 1 stack of 2.

In shower soap dish - 6 Camay, very moist.

On northeast corner of tub - 1 Pears, slightly used.

On northwest corner of tub - 6 Camay in 2 stacks of 3.

Please ask Sophie when she services my room to make sure the stacks are neatly piled and dusted. Also, please advise her that stacks of more than 4 have a tendency to tip. May I suggest that my bedroom window sill is not in use and will make an excellent spot for future soap deliveries?

One more item... I have purchased another bar of bath-sized Imperial Leather which I am keeping in the hotel vault in order to avoid further misunderstandings.

D. Jones

---

**About the author**
*This story has been doing the rounds for many years. The editors would like to thank the elusive Mr Jones for sharing his agony with us and also Pat and David Green for passing the story on.*

---

# SILVERY THREADS

## Adapted by Eiona Roberts (2007)

When we bought our new car last summer, we discovered that a tiny money spider had made a home deep inside the crevices and joints of the driver's wing mirror. Each morning, my husband would clean away the delicate, silvery thread which it had woven overnight across that mirror. However by the following morning a new web had quietly appeared to take the place of the destroyed one.

We later toured Dorset in that car for a whole week and the spider travelled with us, with my husband having to clean away a newly crafted web every morning; in one way it was a shame to destroy such a work of art or a work of nature.

He, assuming the spider was a 'he' and not a 'she', remained inside it until one very windy day we were doing a ton down the M4 when my husband who was driving noticed the spider being flung off into oblivion – or so it seemed.

We thought that the wind had taken him. However the following day we found he'd managed to hang on by the most delicate of threads and had created another new silvery web overnight.

With hindsight, I suppose that that puff of wind which had seemingly blown him away was a trial or challenge for the spider yet he must have been protected by some kind of unseen windshield as well as that delicate thread.

---

We all as people have our emotional storms, winds, trials, etc. but we also have our windshield, if we'd but only allow ourselves to see or feel it. Our personal windshield may be our friends and loved ones; we also have intangible, invisible threads between those whom we love and trust.

When we hold onto those thoughts, or focus on them, we are secure. Should a puff of wind in the form of some kind of crisis come along and catch us unawares, whisking us off course for a while, we can be left floundering. However if we hold on and never lose sight nor grip in our true friends, we can face any trial hurtling our way no matter how big or small it may be.

# THE SHOPPING LIST

## By John Lake (2006)

"And bloody well hurry up!" The words smacked into the back of Derek's head as he shut the door and ventured out into the cold, black, winter's night. As he broke into a run, he went over the list in his head: Twenty number six, a box of matches, and a pint of milk, and ask Fred the shopkeeper if she could borrow five pounds. Tell him she would settle up on Friday as usual. He wasn't allowed to write the list down, but woe betides him if he forgot anything. Derek hated asking Fred for money, but when his step-mum spoke, all the kids listened, and obeyed. At eleven years old, Derek was in no position to argue.

The streets were deserted and Derek sped up. He didn't like the dark and as he ran he started to hum Onward Christian Soldiers... A hymn about war. That would scare any monsters or ghosts away. He passed the Six Bells pub. There was a pitch black, dingy, alley alongside. He remembered the time when once, as he passed by, two men had thrown a coat over his head. He'd been scared lots of times before. His step-mum had made him wet himself on more than one occasion. But when that coat turned his world into a dark, sweaty straight jacket, his fear was total. Derek's legs ceased to operate; he tried to scream, but nothing would come out except a tiny, mouse-like squeal.

The men's footsteps got closer; he knew that the spell had to be broken. Every fibre of his body, every ounce of his concentration focused on one final effort. The screech, which emanated from his throat, started his legs pumping. His arms threw off the smelly, tweedy coat that had masked his freedom. He'd escaped; from what, he wasn't sure, but he knew it wouldn't have been good. The laughter from the men gradually faded as he neared the high street. Of course he never told his Dad or his step-mum.

Derek always ran past that alley in the middle of the road now.

"Can I have twenty number six, a pint of milk, and mum said can she borrow five pounds 'til Friday, please?" gasped Derek breathlessly as he burst through the front door of the shop. "O.K." said Fred, "but tell your mum this is the last time." He always said that, and it always made Derek blush. He seemed a nice man, he never shouted or swore. But like many, he must have had a good idea of what it was like for Derek, and his brothers and sisters at home. And like the rest of them, he chose to keep quiet.

Fred handed over a brown paper bag containing the cigarettes, along with a five-pound note. Derek stuffed both into his one remaining useful pocket. He only had two pairs of trousers and, out of the four pockets, there was only one where he couldn't poke his fingers through to his thigh underneath. Mind you, he'd had them for a good few years. The holes in his knees were more of a concern, and the subject of much amusement to his fellow school pupils.

With the pint of milk clutched tightly in his hand, Derek began the run home. As he passed the big scary alley, he suddenly remembered. He felt sick, his heart started to pound more heavily and his legs turned to jelly. But it wasn't the memory of those men. "The matches, I forgot the matches!!"

Derek ran back as fast as he could, but it was too late. The shop lights were out; Fred had locked up for the day. No matter how hard he stared through the glass and willed him to appear in the gloom, he wouldn't materialise.

Derek started to walk home. Suddenly the thought of staying out as long as possible in the dark was more appealing than what was waiting for him on his return. He had forgotten something off the list.

# CROSSROADS

## By John Lake (2006)

Karl was at the crossroads. For him to even realise this was testament to his ability to swim against the tide. He wanted friends, but not at any price and the recommended retail of friendship was his future. Throughout his schooling, Karl had always been bright and willing to learn. But now, at sixteen, it was decision time.

Karl lived with his father, but his mother was of the step variety. His real mum had left when he was six or seven; it was hard to remember. After a few years of having various aunties, his dad had remarried, more for convenience than out of love.

His step-mum had brought three girls of her own along, Karl and his brother made another two, and just for good measure his dad and step-mum had another boy. Throw in a dilapidated council house and a couple of mongrels and there was Karl's stereotypical dysfunctional family. Dad did go out to work but also spent a fair amount of time in the company of Mr Ladbrokes, while his step-mother was a regular at the bingo hall, spending all the housekeeping trying to win it back.

Karl and his brothers and sisters looked after each other. Who else was there? His real mum saw her sons every other weekend and had reported the neglect and abuse, which was as plain as the latest black eyes on their faces. But social services were conspicuous by their apathy and incompetence.

School was an oasis; at least they all got one meal five days a week. He loved to learn, and when immersed in his latest English or History project, Karl managed to forget his troubles for a few minutes. The playground was another matter; in the early years he had to run the gauntlet of both physical abuse and, worse, the vitriolic truths uttered by the other pupils. Being called a tramp was the worst. Whoever made up that sticks and stones poem hadn't a clue. It wasn't his fault he had no uniform or P.E. kit. A teacher had given him detention for having no football boots. Wasn't it their responsibility to find out what was going on at home?

Despite everything, Karl had always known right from wrong; it would be easy for him to conform to society's expectations of him, but he was determined to escape. Even at eleven he had realised education was the key. So, apart from the days when he was kept at home to cater for his step-mum's needs, Karl soaked up as much knowledge as possible. He excelled at everything except maths, which just floated by, stopping just long enough to deposit the essentials.

But Karl wanted to be liked; don't we all? He had started to succumb to the temptations of mixing with the other local kids. Drinking cider, smoking cigarettes and black Lebanese cannabis, which was particularly popular at that time; certainly the spliff to be seen with. He would stay out to the early hours; there was no one to discipline him; all his boundaries were self-drawn. After all, he had bucketfuls of excuses. He really could blame society.

Here he was then, at the crossroads. He glanced over at his gang of friends, scowled at them for one last time, and headed off to the exam room.

# I DON'T FEEL LIKE DANCING

## By Tracey Kesterton (2007)

Five sleepy bodies sat in the corridor, waiting to be let into the Hospital Gym. Well, they weren't actually waiting – they'd be perfectly content to stay in the corridor and natter, but the physiotherapists often had other ideas.

Wilma yawned, stretching her little legs out before her and wiggling her painted toes.

"Is that your attempt to wake up, from the toes upwards?" Nikki asked.

Wilma gave her best 'pretend-offended' gasp. "You've not noticed? I have a new toe-ring! Look!" More toe-wriggling occurred as everybody admired Wilma's rather fabulous toes and their numerous silver rings in all their splendour.

"That's why you're wearing sandals with no socks on in autumn is it?" Nikki commented, and received an elbow thump in response.

"Is Alvin coming today? It's not quite the same without him moaning all morning is it?" Judy laughed. "And I wonder if he's dyed his hair again?"

"Does he dye his hair?" Nikki gasped.

"Yeah, he was getting a few grey hairs coming through and together with him not being able to walk too straight, old ladies kept trying to help him across the road!" Judy giggled.

"And hair dye helps, does it?" Nikki laughed. "I'll have to try that!"

"Well now he just looks young and incompetent, rather than old and incapable..." Wilma said.

Kate the physiotherapist finally stuck her head round the door to try and move her rabble into the gym next door, but Nikki was ready for her.

"Can we have three teas...? Judy – coffee? Three teas, one coffee and a vodka and tonic please."

"AFTER you've done your exercises!" Kate tried to glare sternly, but her lips kept twisting into a smile. They tried this on every week – they should know the answer by now.

"Wow! Wilma – you can have a vodka after!"

"NO – you can have a cup of tea after and be glad of it. Now COME ON."

Five sets of eyes blinked at her, trying to summon the energy to get out of their chairs – or was it their lack of co-ordination again? Either way, movement into the gym was slow.

"Have you ever watched five people with MS all trying to get out of a 3 door car? Is that not exercise enough?" Nikki asked. "Can't we just stay here for an hour and you just bring us our tea afterwards...?" The door to the gym slammed in answer. That was a 'no' then.

~ ~ ~ ~ ~

It sounded like a good idea, having a Hospital Gym especially for people with the same illness – in this case multiple sclerosis. It was a fun kind of illness where your body generally ignored whatever your brain was telling it to do, so why they thought their clients would be able to safely co-ordinate themselves into a one hour gym class was anybody's guess.

They eventually managed to get themselves into the gym, and proceeded to take their socks off very, very slowly. Some would call this killing time, but Kate was wise to their tricks.

"Nikki, WHAT are you doing?"

"I was going to tell Wilma a joke..."

"You CAN tell her a joke and exercise at the same time you know." Nikki tutted and gave her best 'Paddington stare' as she began to wave her arms vigorously.

"And waving your arms is not one of your exercises either!"

Finally the chatter decreased as the exercises increased slightly. They felt they had to look like they were doing something or they wouldn't get their tea afterwards.

After a while of concentrated exercising, Kate's voice woke everybody with a booming shout. "Alice WHO told you to walk backwards on the cross-trainer?"

"The what?"

"The 'Walking Forwards' machine?"

Alice paused mid step and blinked in confusion. She looked desperately at the rest of group for help but they feigned busyness, keeping their heads down and waving assorted limbs in the air. "Um...they told me it would be EASIER if I walked backwards..." she said, hopefully.

"Easier?" Kate gasped. "We're not here for EASY! Walk forwards, woman!" Alice's legs managed to slowly haul the pedals in the opposite direction. Nobody could quite tell whether she was sulking or not and didn't like to ask.

At the sound of a clatter, Wilma glanced up from her cycling, bit her lip to stop the laugh escaping then hurriedly looked down again. Alvin had entered the gym, half an hour late, in his usual haphazard manner.

And enter it he had, wearing a bright, damp t-shirt with the bolshy slogan reading "I'm not pissed, I have MS" printed boldly across the front. Alvin had clearly had enough of people asking him if he was drunk – as if he'd had the chance at that time of the morning. But it was the apparent streak of hair dye adorning his forehead that had led to Wilma's bitten lip. But at least he didn't look old this week – scary, but not old.

"What?" The question seemed directed at anybody who'd noticed his shaky arrival.

"And what time d'you call this?" Nikki bravely held his gaze. "Have you lost your watch again?" she smiled.

"Look! Before you start, I had an encounter with some...water."

"You haven't been synchronized swimming in the canal again?" Wilma couldn't restrain herself. "I told you that doesn't work! You have to keep moving out of the way when a boat comes along – wrecks your routine!"

Alvin sighed in response. "The ground moved. Again. It wasn't my fault the canal boat leapt in front of me!"

"Or you could try NOT walking past the canal every morning?" Judy suggested. "Next time be prepared honey, accommodate the illness. Try a different route, man!"

~ ~ ~ ~ ~

Eventually Nikki managed to challenge gravity and struggle to her feet, getting her legs stiffly moving in the general direction of the 'hand box' – a tin of various implements meant to strengthen hands and encourage feeling in the bits of her that were now numb. The hand box was the other side of the gym – some might even think it had been left there deliberately so somebody would have to go and fetch it.

"We should start a dance troupe you know!" she announced as she headed gingerly across the gym like a virgin ice skater taking to the rink for the first time. "Hey – we should! We could call ourselves the 'Spastic Slappers' – what d'ya think: six people with MS all in a dance troupe?!"

"Would that be safe?" Wilma cackled.

"Course it would!" Nikki was nothing if not positive. "You know most dance troupes have everybody synchronised doing exactly the same things at the same time? Well the beauty of OUR dance group would be we wouldn't NECESSARILY be co-ordinated.....and we may not be all standing at the end either. But that would be the CHARM of our group! What d'you think? Well? Well?"

There was too much laughter to gauge a response, but Nikki took that to be only positive.

~ ~ ~ ~ ~

Unfortunately, some of Nikki's healthy friends weren't quite so keen. There was glee at the idea initially, but after the giggles died down the doubters started.

"But you can't use that word, you know," one commented.

"What, 'Slappers'? They didn't seem to mind..."

"No, 'Spastic' – you can't use that word any more because it's offensive – they've changed it to something else haven't they? So you can't use it."

"But spasticity is one of the major symptoms of MS – what do you suggest we use?"

They had no answer.

~ ~ ~ ~ ~

Yet enthusiasm remained high at the gym, even if their limbs weren't quite so positive. Alvin managed to get a copy of "Top Hat, White Tie and Tails" and Alice managed to get her hands on six top hats – they decided to use walking sticks instead of canes.

"Bev can't stand for long periods, never mind jiggle – should we get her a Zimmer frame instead?" Judy observed.

"You can't wave a Zimmer over your head like you can a walking stick; it's not the same. Bev, could you sit on the big gym ball and bounce the routine?" Wilma was full of ideas.

"My feet don't reach the floor...."

"Well let some of the air out then...."

Teamwork – they'd never been this united since they thought Edna the tea lady had been in a fight. It turned out she'd said she 'had a bite' but the intention to protect their tea lady had been impressive.

They began to work even harder when Kate found a local dance competition being run by the Council – they had a focus and nothing was going to stop them.

~ ~ ~ ~ ~

MS is an unpredictable illness, but to the best of their ability there were six people going to enter a dance competition. They wouldn't be flawless or synchronised; it would feel like they were dancing in water with the weight of water holding them back due to the stiffness in their limbs. Balance was a bit hit and miss, but the intention was there and, if all else failed, they were determined their enthusiasm would carry them through. Stubbornness and defiance were two of the better symptoms.

~ ~ ~ ~ ~

When they arrived at the City Hall for the competition after months of rehearsing, nerves were high. The hall was starting to fill up with people, and all the troupes were backstage getting ready for their dances.

"Where's my ball – has anybody seen my gym ball?" Bev was flapping. It was nowhere to be seen.

"Dunno – can you use a Space Hopper instead?" Alice asked. "My nephew has one in the shed and he doesn't live far away...."

~ ~ ~ ~ ~

But another problem arose before they solved the mystery of the missing gym ball. Kate arrived looking pale and worried.

"I think we have a problem..." she began. Suddenly she had everybody's attention. "The Council wants us to withdraw from the competition."

"Why? We're not that good!" Wilma laughed.

"They think some people in the audience might get upset at disabled people dancing."

"Might? You mean nobody's ACTUALLY complained; they're just banning us IN CASE somebody gets upset?" Wilma frowned.

"Nobody's complained, but the Council says they're not prepared to take the chance..."

~ ~ ~ ~ ~

Bags were slowly packed; top hats were put back in their boxes. Wilma asked whether they wanted to tap-dance out of the hall to make a proper exit, but the corridor was quite narrow and they didn't think they quite had the co-ordination to dance in a straight line.

~ ~ ~ ~ ~

As they reached the car park, Kate came running up to the group brandishing paperwork and a big smile.

"The Council wants to offer their deep apologies for any inconvenience," she puffed, "...and they wanted me to give you these with their compliments!"

"What are they?" Nikki peered at the papers held in Kate's hand.

"Complimentary tickets for the AUDIENCE of the final of the Dance Competition!"

There was no answer to that, and the little dance troupe silently turned and began to get into the parked cars. When they were seated, Alice gave an enormous sigh of defeat.

"I give up. I don't feel like dancing. Not any more..."

Nikki reached over and gave her friend a consoling hug. "How d'you feel about synchronised swimming next year then?" she grinned, a mischievous glint in her eyes. "Can you swim?"

---

**About the author**
*Tracey Kesterton was 41 when she wrote this story in 2005 after attending a real MS Gym, although they never set up a dance troupe as the patients had no sense of rhythm!*
*Diagnosed in 1990, Tracey worked as a Graphic Artist for 20 years until told she now had secondary progressive multiple sclerosis and couldn't continue working any longer. She is divorced and lives in Birmingham.*

---

# BALANCING ACT

## By Julie Phelan (2007)

The transparent walls act like a force field between the parents and the frantic action unfolding in the inner sanctum. From the centre of the privileged bubble a man wearing one of the white coats suddenly stops as he notices the woman's splayed fingers reaching out towards the glass. Why it should take him by surprise is a surprise in itself. Had they *all* forgotten that this tragedy belonged to them too?

~ ~ ~ ~ ~

Joe and Susan Lister were really very average. Average car, average house, average jobs. Moving from day to day, earning just enough for household expenses and saving just enough for the occasional day out. They had fun. They loved each other. More importantly they *liked* each other. So, when Susan had casually looked into a pram that day last June, and peered over the layers of fleecy blankets to meet with a pair of wide, innocent eyes staring directly into her soul, it was not really that much of a surprise when she blurted out, "Joe, I want one!"

"Huh?" said Joe, turning in surprise. "Want what?"

"A baby," she said quietly. "I want us to have a baby."

"You want to talk about this now, do you?" he sighed, facing her.

"Please," she said. "I just feel it's time. And before you say it, I know money would be tight but if we waited till we had enough we would *never* have one."

"That's your sister talking," Joe replied dismissively. "It would be stupid to rush into anything."

"Hardly rushing! I'm thirty-four, Joe. Loads of women have already completed their family by now."

"Is this really important to you?" Joe asked. Susan nodded. "Well, I suppose we had better make a start then!" Joe said grabbing her round the waist. Susan squealed with laughter causing raised eyebrows from other shoppers. She returned his hug.

"Don't expect everything to be a plain sailing though," he warned. "You know the implications."

"I'll go to the clinic and let them know what we are doing," she replied. "I've already read about pregnancy and diabetes. Loads of other women manage, so why can't I?"

Joe nodded but said no more. Susan's health had always been poor. She had been diagnosed with insulin dependent diabetes at the age of just eight and had monitored herself all her life. Even with all the care she took she still had frequent low blood sugars causing her to become disoriented – Joe had lost count of the times he had woken in the night to find her lying next to him, bathed in sweat and oblivious to the world. He had lost count of the times he had forced sugary drinks down her throat, while she lashed out at him. But, he had survived that, and more importantly so had she, so why should he put a stop to a baby?

~ ~ ~ ~ ~

Month after month there was no cause for celebration. Each morning she would rise, cross her fingers and go into the bathroom. And nothing. Then suddenly...something. For this time as she waited for the little blue line to appear – it *did* appear. Breaking into a grin, she ran to the hall and dialled her husband at work.

"It's positive!" she exclaimed, her voice catching in her throat.

"Oh wow!" Joe sounded thrilled, "Well done! Steady though – don't get excited too soon."

"I know that," Susan said.

"Well, do you though? You know you have a far greater chance of miscarriage than a nor......" he caught himself in time "a woman without diabetes."

"I've just got to get the right balance. Just be happy, will you!"

"I am happy, Sue. Really I am. I'm just worried, sweetheart, that's all."

~ ~ ~ ~ ~

Weeks passed and, with an almost defiant refusal to be different from any other mother, Susan remained fit. She felt better than even before. She ate properly, exercised properly and rested. In fact, she felt better than she had in years. Up until now. As she opened the door and threw down her bag, she caught the look of concern in Joe's eyes.

"I'm having an early night," she said in reply to his expression, her face pale.

"How far have you walked?"

"Too far. I'll be okay; I just need to go to sleep."

Susan got changed and haphazardly sloshed some water over her face. She stood staring at her reflection in confusion. There was something she usually did. What was it? Her eyelids drooped. Whatever it was it could wait. She lay down on the bed and within seconds she was asleep.

~ ~ ~ ~ ~

"Susan? Susan?" Tap. Tap. Tap. Tap.

She was starting to feel irritated. *For God's sake let me sleep!*

"Susan? Susan?" Tap. Tap. Tap. Tap.

She lashed out with an arm and felt her hand meet with thick fabric. She squinted at the light shining squarely at her face.

"Turn it off!" she heard herself scream.

"Susan?" Tap.

"No, she's not coming round, Mike."

Susan tried to speak. Tried to tell them she could hear them. She felt a sharp stab into her thigh and heavy pressure as something cool plunged into the muscle. She could hear voices. Woozily she opened her eyes and faces floated in and out of focus.

"Hello, you. Welcome back," Joe smiled. But his smile froze on his face as Susan cried out and gasped.

"Oh my God! It's the baby!"

The sudden flurry of activity created total pandemonium in the bedroom. Paramedics threw instructions at each other. Susan couldn't remember what to do. Confused and disoriented she started to sob quietly.

"Don't get upset!" Joe ordered.

Two men in green stood each side of her and led her slowly through the house and to the back of the waiting ambulance. The siren yelped to herald its departure and Joe jumped in the back and grasped her hand. As the ambulance sped through the streets, her contractions came more and more frequently. The objects around her were still hazy and blurred as her hand tightened around his.

Suddenly the doors of the ambulance flew open and she was lifted off one bed and onto another. The cold air smacked her face as she was wheeled out across the tarmac and then into the bright artificial lights of the accident and emergency. People turned in surprise as the ever-growing cast of actors thundered through the doors to the maternity unit.

Crashing into an empty room, gas and air were thrust onto her face and Susan sucked them in hungrily. Waves of pressure were building greater and greater and then it happened. Too soon. A small bundle of pink flesh slid out onto the sheet.

A nurse dived to the child, cut the cord and carried it away. Time stood still. The room had fallen strangely quiet. Unnervingly quiet. A nurse was pressing on the baby's chest using two fingers and clearing out its mouth. Still no sound. Susan and Joe could do nothing but gaze helplessly at the tiny little form and the sea of hands and tubes that surrounded it.

And then, without a word, the baby was lifted up and taken away. Susan and Joe had been somehow forgotten. Grabbing a gown from the bed, she placed two unsteady feet on the floor.

"What the hell are you doing?" Joe exclaimed.

"Well, I'm not sitting here!" Rising awkwardly to her feet she leant on Joe for support, and together they made their way along the empty corridor. The reception desk was empty but a sign leading to the Neonatal Intensive Care Unit was clear enough.

"Down there. Come on," she urged.

The short corridor led into an area with huge windows overlooking two rooms filled with cots. Each cot was hooked up to wires, monitors and plastic tubes. And inside the cots small bodies lay immobile attached to equipment that flashed with green lights.

"Oh, look at them all!" Susan gasped.

Looking across the sea of little cots they saw a further glass room beyond. The restless movement of white coats exuded a certain desperation that accompanied any uncertain attempt at a miracle. And today that attempt would be the little life of Ellie. Susan and Joe watched transfixed as doctors mimed orders to each other and directed nurses to equipment.

Then as suddenly as the panic had started it stopped. The nurses' hands slowed, the doctor looked at his watch and wrote something down on a chart.

Susan held her breath and reached out with one hand towards the glass. He turned with surprise to see them standing there. Looking straight at them, he placed the clipboard down, enabling him to raise both hands with thumbs pointing upwards as he mouthed "Okay!"

They hadn't been forgotten after all.

# A TALE OF TWO

## By Lianne Potts (2007)

"DDRRIIIINNNGGG!"

The Neo-school bell rang, almost deafening Alex, when 1,000 Neopets stormed inside like a herd of Blurgahs, as well as trampling Alex flat as Blumaroo pancakes. When the playground was eventually deserted, the rather worn out (not to mention squashed) Acara slowly pulled himself off the ground while dusting down his trousers. There was no harm done to him at all, though. This was a daily routine to Alex!

The Acara was eventually inside the Neo-school himself, trying at least to avoid the Techos and Jub-Jubs rushing one way, and the Shoyrus and Kougras dashing the other, who were late, like Alex. He zipped over as quickly as he could along the corridor that seemed to never end, until he reached his destination. Class 5B. As the breathless Acara opened the creaking door, he heard the horribly familiar voice of Mrs Moehog, moaning:

"Alex Acara! This is the fourth time you've been late for class this week! Detention!"

"B-but Mrs Moehog," Alex tried to explain urgently, "the Altador Cup..."

"Oh, that stupid game," whined the grumpy 5B teacher. "I don't care. Sit down at the back. NOW!"

Alex plodded gloomily to the back of the classroom, head hanging. But, to his relief, there to brighten his day a little was Max. Max was Alex's closest friend. In fact his only friend, come to think of it. Everyone else called him "Custard Face" and "Useless Yellow Furball". They also teased Alex about the size of his ears, and said they were girly. So, the only person at school the lonely Acara could rely on, was Max. The only problem was that Max was sometimes a big, mean and nasty, bully.

After his usual boring day at Neo-school (well, all boring except break), something dawned on Alex. Detention. Stupid, rubbish detention. With a displeased groan, Alex was on his way to dreaded detention. Who invented detention any way? Whoever they were, they must have been pretty evil, huh? I mean, what's the point in sitting in a silent and dusty room like a ghost Meepit anyway?

To Alex's surprise, there to put his mind off the boredom, and the fact he was missing a really great game, was Max. What a relief! The Acara pulled out a chair, and whispered:

"Hey Max! What are you doing in here?"

"Huh? What? Oh, hey Alex! What you in here for, then? Tripping people up with your ears too often?" teased Max.

"No, you know perfectly well. I was late in 4 times in a row. And, like I said, why are you here?"

"Me? Oh, I stole the Gummy Gems off all the Kaus in 3A," Max admitted cheerfully, although inside he was very ashamed.

"Hey, you two! The Meerca and Acara! No talking in the detention room!" Mr Scorchio bellowed louder than Sloth. No-one messes with him!

The next bright and beautiful Neopian morning at 09:00 NST, Alex finally managed to avoid all the Neo-school rush completely! He was so pleased he had finally achieved one of his biggest targets! After his moment of victory, on the way to his locker, Alex suddenly stumbled into Max. Max had some news, although Alex didn't seem to like it very much. It was that it was Maths with Miss Eyrie first thing.

"Oh, nuts!" Alex groaned with dread in his sky blue eyes.

After what seemed like ages of pure boredom with Miss Eyrie, Max leaned over to Alex and whispered:

"Hey, that detention with Mr Scorchio wasn't all that bad, was it?"

"Really? You think so? Well, I'm scared of him. Are you?"

"Ha! No way, wimpy! You're a real weed!"

Alex could not believe his ears. His best friend, his only friend, calling him a wimp! A weed! Alex knew Max was a bit of a meanie, but this had gone too far. This was it!

At lunch that terrible, terrible day, Alex sat at the very back of the lunch hall, only poking at his Broccoli and Cheese Pizza. Alex was alone on his table, until along came one of the Kaus, who looked sorry for the poor Acara. She sat down beside Alex and sympathetically said:

"Hey, what's up Mr Grumpy-Face?"

"Nothing. Now if you don't mind I would prefer to be alone," Alex grumbled.

"Aw, c'mon! I won't blab. Promise! Do I sound like a scammer?" the Kau re-assured the lonely Acara beside her.

"OK. It's Max. He's my only friend, and now he's calling me a weedy wimp! Some friend."

"It's alright. I know what he's like. He stole all of my and my friends' Gummy Gems!" the Kau exclaimed.

When Alex left the lunch hall that sunny Friday afternoon, he was feeling a lot like the sun: bright and cheery. It made him feel good that someone else felt like him now.

At 15:00 NST, Alex zoomed to his Neo-home on his favourite Droolik scooter, dumped his Jeran backpack on his Walking Carpet Rug, and flopped into his Red Bean Bag. Then, it dawned on Alex. What was Max feeling like? Was he grinning away happily, lying on his Orange Jelly couch, and thinking:

'Ha ha! That was so good, making Alex upset. I bet he's in his room crying his head off! Mumsie, that meanie Max is horrible! I want my Bruce Plushie! Waah! He-he-he!'

Nah. He was Alex's only friend, and he would never leave him. Alex thought that it would be more likely that he was thinking:

'I shouldn't have made Alex feel bad. He might not want to be friends with me anymore, and then he'll be alone in Neopia! Oh, what've I done?'

And Alex was right. Max was curled up with his Florg Plushie, and saying to himself:

"I didn't mean to upset him. It just popped out of my mouth. I can't help being a big meanie; it's just me, it's who I am! Oh man, what do I do? Well, you would just eat the nearest thing, wouldn't you, Florgy? Oh, gosh. I have to apologise. I would never live it down."

The next day was brighter than before and also both Max and Alex's favourite day: Saturday! No school, no homework, and definitely no Miss Eyrie blabbing on about the 7 times table! That morning, when Alex was just about to go out and play with his friends, he noticed his calendar. The Month of Relaxing! Yessss! After all that waiting, it was finally there – The Altador Cup! That brought back so many memories to Alex. Autrey Fulse passes one Faerielander, then another, Valtonos Rea gets ready, dives, but it's another point for the Haunted Woods team! The crowd goes wild! YEEAAAHH!!

This reminded Alex of his 'friend' Max. Last year, they had front row seats, a Jelly Slushie each, and smiles on their faces, as their favourite team stormed to victory! Some of the happiest memories that sprung into Alex's mind were Max spilling his Slushie all over the Koi in front of them, and they both almost got sent back to their Neo-homes when a security guard saw Max booing because the Lost Desert team scored a goal!

"Whoa, that was fun. Wish I knew if can trust you or not, pal," sighed Alex as he gazed out of his window, eyes fixed on Max's Neo-home.

Alex logged on to his laptop, when almost instantly there was a message at the top of the screen. It read: 'You have neo-mail!'

"That's odd," thought Alex. "I never get neo-mail. Hang on. Maybe it's Max! We can be friends again!"

And with that, the button was clicked. And Alex was right! It was from Max. It read:

"Hello Alex! I am so sorry I called you a weedy wimp. I don't know what came over me. To apologise, I've spent all the Neopoints in my Snorkle money tin to buy us a ticket each to see Haunted Woods vs. Virtupets next Saturday. Wanna come?

From Max :>)"

Now Max and Alex are still friends to this day, even though the occasional argument pops up every now and then, isn't that right you two?

**About the author**
*Lianne Potts is 10 years old and is in Year 6 at Primary School in the Royal County of Berkshire. She totally loves reading and writing stories on just about anything that interests her. One of her main interests at the moment is the totally fantastic new series of Doctor Who and she's kind of idolising Russell T. Davies. The awesome BBC Doctor Who website has a Comic Maker section where Lianne's imagination can run wild creating story lines and graphics for her own imaginary episodes. Other interests are creating animations using plasticine and most star "Blue Person" in short 2 minute films of highjinks and fun. And Beano comics – say no more!*
*Watch out world, here comes LIANNE.............*

# EASTER BREAK

## By Anthony Webster (2007)

You'd have thought that, at their age, we could have left them for half an hour while we walked the dogs together. But no. What do we find when we get back home? The pair of them standing in the kitchen, looking sheepish. We immediately knew there was something wrong.

"What's the matter?" I asked, in a flat, matter-of-fact tone of voice; nothing accusatory about it at all.

"We weren't even here when it happened," responded one hastily, "were we?"

"No, we were in the sitting room playing cards," added the other.

After all my years in the teaching profession, I'm well used to the excuse routine, so I suppose I could have gone into automatic pilot mode at that point.

"Well, what happened?" I enquired with a resigned tone in my voice, "You'd better tell me all about it – from the beginning."

"It's one of the geese, smashed to smithereens on the floor," began one.

"It must have been in a thousand pieces. They were so small it took us ages to pick them up," added the other.

The sense of exaggeration was clear but I looked upward, above the cooker hood, to where my small porcelain collection of mother goose and her four goslings have happily sat, surveying their kitchen scene, for years. Except now there was a gap.

"Well, if you weren't in here, how do you think it happened?" I asked. "Porcelain geese don't suddenly take to flying after years on their perch, do they? And they certainly don't commit hara-kiri!"

"We think it must have been the cats," said one. "They both scurried out of here when we came in, didn't they?"

"Yes," affirmed the other, "there was a great clatter, so we came rushing in. Have they climbed up there before?"

"Never!" I retorted somewhat abruptly. I think they both got the message that I was finding this tale a bit hard to swallow; the idea of either of those two rushing anywhere was quite ludicrous in itself.

"Anyway," I continued, "I wouldn't have expected a huge noise from a porcelain gosling, no matter how many pieces it broke into."

"We thought that, as well," said one, "but it's all we found."

My incredulity was being stretched to its extreme but then, as my eyes scanned the full width of the tops of the wall units, I noticed that one of the decorative enamel saucepans I keep up there was at a precarious angle – and its lid was missing. They, of course, had both followed my gaze, and there was an air of triumph in their eyes as they focused on that pan. Soon the errant lid, no doubt the author of the din which had attracted them from their game of cards in the first place, was retrieved from amongst the cutlery on the draining board. I had to admit to myself that neither of them was able to get up there and dislodge a saucepan, so the cat story would have to be accepted, at least for now.

But we'll think twice before leaving the pair of them home alone again. Having both our mothers staying in the house at the same time was causing more problems than we'd anticipated.


# TAXI DRIVER

## By Sam Meldrum (1999)

I never did like that Maggie Thatcher you know, but you've gotta admire her haven't you? And that John Major, well, I can't understand that, well, I don't think anyone can. Now, Tony Blair he seems alright, but his ears are all wrong. If he wants to be a really successful leader he'll just have to get them pinned. Same goes for Charlie boy really. That son of his, William, though, he's none of his father's shortcomings, you mark my words, he'll have no problem keeping hold of a good lady.

Ian Beale and that Melanie, who'd have thought it?

Still Princess Di, too good for him so she was. And that Harry, well, I'd get those ears pinned before it's too late, those school chums of his will be giving him grief. He'll never be able to live up to the playboy image of the second-in-line if they leave it too late. Scar a man for life something like that, well, I should know, no, it's not the ears, it's well... it's obvious really, innit? And all that nonsense when

Diana passed on, overblown sentimentality if you ask me. 'Course, I cried for a week non-stop. But then, I knew her right, 'cos she came to our school when I was just a nipper and out of all the kids there she came and asked me if I liked it there. Probably 'cos of my... well, you know. I had a bit of trouble getting anything out, see I was shy then, not that you'd know it now.

And that last train, what a load of old nonsense, see if I was in charge I'd know what to do, got to go about repopulating the planet haven't you. Everyone knows that. Seen it a million times at the flicks. And that scientist lass is asking for it if you ask me.

Now, don't talk to me about pop music.. it's just not the same as it were when I was a lad. We had ABBA y'know. Proper music we had.

They should bring back hanging, that's what I says to the missus. Chop the balls off them rapist types. I'll tell you this for nothing, those Arabs have got that right y'know. Now I'm not saying I agree with the way they treats their women mind. Disgraceful, all them foreign religions where they have to cover themselves up and gets married off at fourteen. Dirty buggers the lot of them. Now, Maggie agrees with me there you know, capital punishment, she was all for it. Let them show a bit of flesh, get rid of them silly black veil things, some of them can be quite attractive underneath all that kafuffle. That's what I say anyways.

Now, nuns. What's all that about? Good, honest hard working women depriving themselves. Let me tell you what they need...

Oh here we are love, Paddington Station, that'll be £7.90 please.

Thanks very much darlin'.

Much appreciated. You take care now.

~ ~ ~ ~ ~

Bit of a looker she was. Had her eating out of the palm of my hand. 'Course, she would've been up for it, but I gotta earn a living right?

~ ~ ~ ~ ~

Yes guv. Shepherds Bush. No problem, hop in.

**About the author**
*Sam Meldrum lives in Buckinghamshire with his wife and two young daughters.*

# ON THE MOUNTAIN

## By Natasha Cowan (2007)

One day a girl called Aimee got sick. She was always a loving, beautiful and caring girl.

Later that day a doctor came to her house, and she had tests done. She was later diagnosed with MS.

MS is a horrible thing to have so we, as her friends, went to visit her the next day. We brought Aimee some presents, cards and a big bunch of sunflowers.

Aimee was looking a lot better, but not feeling better. Everything seemed to be happening so fast to her.

Aimee said thank you for the wonderful things we brought her. A while later Aimee's mum came to the room and said it was getting late, and Aimee needed to rest. We gave Aimee hugs and kisses and said goodnight, and we would visit again tomorrow.

The next day as promised, we went to visit Aimee, but we were not allowed in as Aimee had taken really sick overnight. The doctor had been with Aimee since 2 a.m. and was still there at 8 a.m.

We called back that evening to visit Aimee. I asked her, "What have you always dreamt of doing?" Aimee's reply was: "I have always dreamt of climbing a mountain." So we left for the evening to allow Aimee to rest.

We booked a tour of climbing the highest mountain.

Later that week, we left for the tour to the mountain. We all climbed it together; slowly but surely we got to the top safely.

We were so hungry and thirsty when we got to the top. Luckily I had packed snacks and drinks for us. We rested, and then started the descent off the mountain.

Aimee started to say she felt better. Of course we didn't believe her at first. Once we got to the bottom of the mountain Aimee started jumping up and down and skipping around the place. It was like a miracle had happened.

We phoned our parents and told them, they came rushing over to pick us up.

They couldn't believe the change in Aimee, and we celebrated. We went out later that night for a Chinese. It was wonderful.

The doctor called to see Aimee later. He told her she had made a recovery but warned her that the fight wasn't over yet.

Aimee has never fully recovered but, 22 years since that night, Aimee still lives a happy life, with 2 wonderful children and a great husband.

So for those of you with MS, your miracle could be waiting just around the corner, so don't go down without a fight.

---

**About the author**
*Natasha Cowan wrote this touching story at the age of 11, when she saw how difficult everyday tasks had become for her mother, Jacqui. Natasha hopes to carry on writing short stories and would like to help raise funds for research into multiple sclerosis.*

---

# GRANDMOTHER, CIDER AND TALES

## By Zoe Kirkby (2007)

Louise felt the stony silence in the kitchen. It hung cold around her shoulders as she plunged plate after plate into the sink of hot, bubbly water. Rose, her mother, sat at the table nursing a freshly brewed coffee. Louise had no sympathy as she had watched her mother nurse a sore head and reluctantly force a bowl of porridge down earlier.

As the last plate slipped into the draining tray, Louise turned, her hands still dripping soapsuds over the tiled floor.

"Mother, I wish you didn't behave so ... well... you know. Get so drunk when the children are around." Louise had moved in with her parents shortly after her diagnosis. It worked well: Louise was a single parent; her mother helped with the children when Louise had a bad day.

"Nonsense, I was only tipsy. Are you saying I should not enjoy myself?" Rose said, folding her arms across her chest, frowning.

"No, no that is not what I meant." Louise dried her hands and looked at the floor.

"Actually, I think that is exactly what you meant;" excused Rose, "you do not like the thought of me going out, especially now your father's gone." Louise's father had died only a couple of months before.

"It isn't that, mother," Louise sat down to face her. "It's just...well...it's like you have forgotten dad, you're acting as if he never existed."

"That's rubbish and you know it." Rose stood up, hurt.

"No mother, I don't, and you give me no reason to think otherwise."

"Now you listen to me," Rose jabbed her forefinger towards her daughter. "I will not be spoken to like this, do you hear? I am doing what your father never let me do: live my life, meet new people and, yes, that means going out, but it doesn't mean I have forgotten your father."

"And getting drunk?" snapped Louise.

"Well yes OK, perhaps I have had the odd one or two too many. I admit it, but what would you prefer, me shrivelled up in that corner chair, like I used to be?" She paused to sit again and looked at her daughter. "With your father gone, I can be me again. I know that sounds harsh, but you know how things stood around here back then."

Louise felt swamped with guilt and just nodded. She had never been aware of her father's aggressive side, not until she had moved in. He never hit anyone; he just manipulated and twisted things so that he controlled every situation. Her mother could not even go to the shops without giving a full detailed report. She had to explain who she had spoken to, where she had gone and how much she had spent.

Louise ignored this at first, waited to see if her father tried it with her; he did not. Therefore, she raised the subject with her mother after a few weeks. The discussion was short lived. Rose had merely fobbed her off with some excuse about it being her father's way.

Now, seeing the way her mother had exploded into life since his death, she could not help feeling guilty. If only she had spoken to her father, made him see how controlling he was being, maybe things would have been nicer for them all in the end. Even in death, he had controlled the house with iron rule until recently.

The previous night, Louise's children had witnessed their grandmother arriving home drunk. They thought it was hilarious. She had tripped on the mat, fallen through the door and had burst into fits of giggles. The children wafted their hands in front of their faces as sharp cider fumes filled the hall. After guiding Rose into the lounge, they had sat eyes bright and mouths agape as Rose proceeded to tell them the most bizarre stories. Louise just rolled her eyes at her children and left the room.

"Look love," Rose rested her hand on her daughter's, "I know this is hard, but I have not forgotten your father, whatever it looks like. It is just I feel free again, but I can see that I have acted irresponsibly, I should've thought. Let's leave it at that; I promise it won't happen again."

Louise put her smooth hand on top of the ageing one and squeezed. "It's okay mum, I just panicked that's all. What if I needed you in the night?"

"I would have been there."

"What, breathing cider fumes over everyone and giggling like a little girl? Yes, that would've been a great help," said Louise, her shoulders jiggling as she tried to control the laughter before it spilled.

Rose swiped her hand across her forehead in a joke-like manner. "Phew, thought I was going to be grounded for a week," she said, before laughing her infectious laugh, as the embarrassing flashbacks of the night before became all too clear.

---

**About the author**
*Zoe Kirkby was 32 when she wrote this story in 2007. She was diagnosed with scoliosis in her twenties and lives in Somerset with her son. Zoe has a keen interest in family history and developed a passion for writing after studying with the Open University.*

---

# MUMMY THE FAIRY

## Part I by Emily Carter Gibson (2002)

Once upon a time there was a mummy.

One day mummy was sat on her computer when some nutter from the internet started talking to her. Mummy got very excited about this and started talking to the nutter via the powers that be. The nutter liked mummy so much that she said mummy could be a fairy. Mummy got very overexcited about this because mummy had always thought she had special powers. She was even more excited when she got a special magazine for fairies called Fairy Tales. It had Charlie Dimmock in it. She didn't wear a bra either.

One day mummy was walking her skanky dog through some woods when she saw a little green man. He was wearing some suede pixie shoes and a beige corduroy body warmer. Mummy liked the little green man so much she called him Harry and took him back to her castle in the clouds. She showed him her special fairy wings and her fairy smock that she had to wear when performing her special fairy rituals with her special fairy powers.

Sometimes mummy would use her special rocks that she dug up from the ground. She would sell the rocks to gypsies. The gypsies liked the rocks very much because they made them feel all giddy. Harry liked the rocks too. Harry wanted to be a fairy so mummy trained him using the Fairy Handbook Guide to Training Pixies to Become Fairies (this is available to buy at all good fairy shops for just twelve special rocks).

The fairy Queen thought mummy was doing so well that she deserved a promotion to Head of Advertising at the Fiftieth Official Fairy Convention. The convention was to be held in mummy's castle so she scattered rocks everywhere to make it extra super special for all the extra super special fairies. The convention was so good that mummy became Deputy Queen of the Fairies and Harry was her pixie-in-waiting.

Mummy lived happily ever after with Daddy (who disapproved of the fairyness at first but secretly liked the outfits). Mummy always was 'special'.

## Part II by Elizabeth Newlands (2002)

Mummy, dressed in pale blue dungarees (her fairy work and skanky dog walking clothes), had earlier felt the rocks and knew that this day would leave lasting memories for her and those close to her, but how was it to be special, she mused, as she strolled pooper bag at hand.

"If only I wasn't one rock short of a full complement I would know," she thought, but then, "Que sera sera," as her normal thoughts (as opposed to fairy) returned and she continued on her way unperturbed on this crisp morning. There were dapples of sunlight showing through the trees and suddenly, as if by magic, she spied the bollards ahead.

Mummy was urged on remembering her childhood and those endless cross stitch samplers. No one was around: she could realise her childhood desire to leapfrog (recognised fairylike tendencies). Could this be what the rocks had foretold that morning? Oh, if only she had that extra one!

In a world of her own, her fairylike body tingling with anticipation, she positioned herself for the leap, as her shoeless feet left the ground, her wings drawn back in a funnel of wind, her braless form knew only the ecstasy of near fulfilment (sorry if you find this offensive) as she went for the leap, but then, disaster struck. Mummy suddenly found herself dangling, her limbs outstretched, as she remembered too late that her dungarees were of the low slung crotch design for longer bodied women.

At that moment, as if by fairy (and rock) magic, along came the little green man who, realising Mummy's dilemma, eased her solicitously off the bollard and she continued on her way.

## Part III by Emily Carter Gibson (2002)

One sunny day Mummy was walking her skanky dog. She was having such a jolly lovely time, jumping over bollards and reciting angel songs. However, disaster was soon to strike. She bent down to carefully pick up one of the skank's deposits in a folded-up Morrison's bag, but she stood up too quickly, hitting her halo on a rather low branch. She fell to the ground, legs akimbo, dog crap flying (alas, she didn't have time to tie up the bag into a neat bow, ensuring the safe and environmentally friendly decomposition of the excrement).

As luck would have it, Daddy (who had had his fairy privileges removed when he tried to sell Mummy's best gold halo) came skipping along the path and came across Mummy who was still lying, bedraggled, in the mud. Daddy, what with his bad back, was unable to carry Mummy back home so had to go and fetch his best wheelbarrow (no-one else could have done this, since you had to have a licence to drive a wheelbarrow) from his shed.

They were nearly home when they encountered another problem: the step to go inside the house was too large, how would they get Mummy inside? But the Powers That Be had witnessed the whole incident, and magically flew Mummy inside the house. Mummy was soon surrounded once again by her rocks and crystals which ensured a quick recovery. She was also rewarded with a new halo for her bravery.

Mummy, however, got a bit over-excited by all this, and had to go to the toilet. She thought she would be able to walk there but as she got up out of bed her leg buckled – she had tragically pulled her hamstring. A hot water bottle and a bag of frozen peas later, Mummy was walking again.

At first she could only walk around on tip-toes, but after she had sprinkled some fairy dust, rubbed herself down with some healing colours and inhaled some crystals, she could float around the house like a proper angel. Mummy was a very brave fairy indeed.

---

**About the authors**
*Mummy the Fairy was originally an exchange of e-mails following Emily's mother being made an honorary fairy by a fairy believers group (or something like that).*
*Emily is at university studying fashion. She has won awards for her creativity. She has an elderly cat that lives at home with her parents.*
*Elizabeth Newlands was rather hoping to have one of her odes published too but being a friend of one of the editors really doesn't help because we ran out of space so chopped it. Had we published the ode, Elizabeth would have thanked all those who made it possible: her late parents, teachers, husband, friends, and the hula hoops factory (it made sense with the ode, honest) and finally her computer. Elizabeth lives with her husband in leafy Surrey. She does not have any pets. Her hobbies include going out, having fun and holidays.*

---

# THE NEAREST W.C.

## By Anon

A newly married couple viewed a house in the country and decided to buy it. After arriving home they suddenly remembered that they did not know where the W.C. was, so they wrote to the vicar (who had shown them over the place) and asked him if he knew just where it was. The vicar, being ignorant of the term W.C., thought that they meant the Wesleyan Chapel, so imagine their surprise on receiving this letter:

*Dear Sir*

*In reply to your letter, the nearest W.C. I know in the area is 7 miles from the house. This is rather unfortunate if you are in the habit of going regularly. However some people take their lunch and make a day of it. Those who can spare the time walk, others go by train and usually manage to get there in time.*

*By the way, it is made to seat 200 and the council have decided to have plush seats installed to ensure greater comfort. The last time my wife went she had to stand the whole time – I myself never go.*

*There are special facilities for young ladies presided over very kindly by the curate who goes to their assistance when required, and the children sit together and sing during the procedure.*

*Hoping that this will be of great use to you*

*Yours faithfully*

*R.B. Winterbottom*

*P.S. Hymn sheets are provided and will be found hanging near the door.*

---

**About the author**
*The author of this amusing tale is unknown, as is whether the tale is a work of fiction or based in fact. The editors would like to thank Pat and David Green for passing it on for your enjoyment.*

---

# BETTER TO LIVE THAN DREAM...

## By Bianca Wilding (2007)

Neptune had always been Judy's passion. She loved space and planets, and in her dreams she always thought of visiting there. But Judy's dreams always seemed to be too far out of this world. Every single time she dreamed about space and the dazzling stars that shone above in the night sky, they were always washed away by the sound of her boss, Mrs. Longrench, shouting and cursing.

Judy was a junior chef in the local seafood restaurant called 'Seaby Seafood'. But Judy could never concentrate on the pots and pans. Neptune always consumed her thoughts. That or Mrs. Longrench's bellowing voice telling Judy, "That needs more attention" or "Chuck that away: it's burnt." Mrs. Longrench wanted her 'fantastic' restaurant to keep a high reputation. Hardly anybody ever visited!

Finally, 10.30 p.m. arrived. Closing time. Time for Judy to go home. She took off her hat and apron, grabbed her coat and fled to the bus-stop.

Judy's home was a modest flat situated on the second floor facing the local library. She turned her key in the lock and walked through the front door. It was black; pitch black. She reached for the light switch and switched it on. As her eyes adjusted to the light, Judy turned around to find an old man standing opposite her. Judy froze with fear.

"Don't panic, me love," said the very strange looking intruder. His voice was grating, and his grey moustache bobbed up and down as he spoke.

"Wh-Who are you? Get out of my house n-now!" Judy stuttered, looking the man up and down. He had a long skinny face with a huge, shiny button nose. His hair was bushy and dirty, his clothes were tatty and filthy, and he seemed not to be wearing any shoes. Two abnormally large feet stood there on Judy's spotless floor.

"I can't go. I'm Stoomcha. Can't tell me to go, ya know!" Stoomcha replied, shrugging his skinny shoulders. "Everything will be explained. Please calm down," he said in a higher-pitched voice.

"That is easy for you to say. I come into my home, to find an old man standing in it. Why?!" Judy replied, almost screaming.

"Look, I know this is upsetting for you, but please hear me out. If you're not impressed, call the police. Do we have a deal?"

So (through gritted teeth) Judy listened. Stoomcha explained that he was a 'wizariamite', and that he was here to grant Judy a wish. He retold a memory of Judy's from when she was only twelve.

"Do you remember when you wrote down a specific wish that you sent on a balloon? Well, us wizariamites hide in the clouds and we make people's wishes come true. Only for people who deserve it, of course," Stoomcha explained using big hand expressions.

"My goodness, I remember that. My wish was to go to Neptune. But wait! If you are this 'wizariamite', then why did you leave it till now to grant me my wish? That was years ago!" Judy replied, holding her hips.

"I was just waiting for the time when you most needed it. Your work is dragging you down, and you're in a little old flat on your own. So now is best time to visit good ol' Neptune, eh?" Stoomcha gave Judy a knowing wink.

Judy thought long and hard and finally said, "I've decided to go along with your little wizariamite thing, but if this is some sort of joke it's only three numbers away from the police," Judy said, grabbing the phone. "But, yes, I accept," she added.

As Stoomcha was about to wave his wand, Judy's cat, Chuggles, came in. He was hissing and scratching towards Stoomcha.

"Ah, perfect. Watch this Judy."

"Bad manners, you silly cat, from bad to good. Be quick with that!" sang Stoomcha. Green and gold sparks shot from the wand and formed a circle around Chuggles. Chuggles lifted off the ground, slowly spun once, and then landed again.

To prove that the spell had worked, Stoomcha summoned Chuggles. When he did, Chuggles pounced over and brushed his leg against Stoomcha's leg, purring as loud as he ever had

"My goodness!" Judy cried. "Chuggles would never do that!"

"Well, my magic does work then, don't it my love! But anyways, let's get back to the point. Neptune..." Stoomcha was cut short.

"How are you going to get me to Neptune?" Judy interrupted, frowning.

"Let me finish. I'll teleport you there using my wand. I think you'll love Neptune. When you come back, all ya gotta do is spin around three times and say 'Seaby, Seaby, Seaby'. Got that?" he said, fiddling with his twig-like wand.

"Seaby three times? Well, OK, I'm ready," said Judy, putting her trainers on.

"Judy, Neptune, Judy, Neptune, Judy, Neptune," shouted Stoomcha and, once again, green and gold sparks shot out of the wand and formed a large circle around Judy. VWOOSH. She was spinning. Fast, which felt like an eternity but just as she started to get afraid, she was there. Neptune. She fell to the ground, as she was so terribly dizzy.

Once Judy's head had recovered she took a long look around. The scenery was amazing. The sky was a turquoise blue. The ground was smooth and shiny; a soft magnolia colour, it looked like marble. Towering rocks that looked like some sort of castle stood before her. It would be stupid not to see inside having come this far, so off she ran. As she came closer, the rocks were bigger than Judy had expected. But she was fearless and explored further. Suddenly she heard a noise she had never heard before.

"Hello? Hello? Who's there? Stoomcha?" Judy's eyes widened and her jaw dropped. Before her stood something phenomenal.

Judy was looking at a very unique creature. Its body was pear-shaped and scaly. A greeny colour. Two long blue antennae were on top of its head, and one yellow eye stuck out in the middle of its forehead. Judy didn't know what to think. Was it friendly? Was it a killer? All Judy did know was that she was the first person to ever discover a new creature from a different planet.

"Migalominoshlya," the creature gargled.

Stoomcha suddenly appeared in a nanosecond flash. Judy flinched.

"Ah, so you've finally found a Neptarlian!" Stoomcha grinned.

"A Neptarlian, wow, really? Is it friendly?" questioned Judy, playing nervously with her hair.

"This one's friendly: it has green scales. It's those reduns you gotta stay away from!" said Stoomcha mysteriously.

"Why? What will they do?" Judy asked, biting her fingernails.

"Well, you might get hypnotised, but most likely you'll be knocked unconscious then turned into a spec of dust on the Neptune floor. Fancy that?"

"Umm, no thanks. I'll keep a look out for those," sighed Judy, running her skinny fingers through her long, curly hair once again.

"Well, I must be off now. Bysie-bye." Stoomcha waved goodbye and dissolved into the air.

So Judy still carried on her adventure to the castle of rocks. She walked closer and closer, towards the Neptarlian.

"Hello, do, you want me, to go, in, there?" Judy tried to say using an easy sign language.

"LapLaptungimiglyashynaa," it replied directing Judy into the Castle.

I'll take that as a 'yes' then, Judy thought.

Inside this strange castle was something Judy could never have imagined. Long lines of rope hung from the ceiling, moving in the light breeze. Golden statues of Neptarlians stood everywhere around the massive room. But there, in the middle of the room, stood steps to a throne where an ancient Neptarlian was seated. Its antennae were yellow instead of blue; its eye was green instead of yellow. But worst of all, its scales were red. This Neptarlian was obviously the king.

"TANLACKSTOVIMIGLOYANASH," screamed the king, standing up from his throne and flying towards Judy. Judy didn't say a word, she just ran for her life.

Judy was soon out of breath, and she had a stitch so bad that tears rolled down her cheeks. She quickly turned back to find the Neptarlian close enough to reach out and touch. She knew what was going to happen, but she just couldn't run anymore. All she saw were two yellow antennae coming towards her, and then she went deathly cold and started to shake. Everything went black. Judy had been knocked out by a red Neptarlian.

Judy awoke looking at a familiar ceiling. White swirls on it. Yes. It was the ceiling of Judy's flat. She sat up looking at her front door. Just at that moment, Stoomcha burst through the door.

"Stoomcha, I'm so glad to see you. Please help me! Is the Neptarlian here? Get rid of it. I'm so glad I'm alive, aren't I?" sobbed Judy, clinging onto Stoomcha's arm.

"You are alive, and you're lucky to be. It's also lucky that I turned up when I did. Cuz' you would have died if I hadn't," replied Stoomcha in a lower voice.

"Thank you for Sa-"

"Oh, there's no need to thank me, believe me!" he interrupted, with a disturbing look on his face. Just as he said that, he evaporated into the air, leaving a small stone behind. A stone of Neptune. Judy kept this on her mantelpiece for the rest of her life, although she was loath to touch it. It was her souvenir from her once most favourite place in the whole universe. Neptune. She never dreamed of going back.

---

**About the author**
*Bianca Wilding, who is 12 years of age, hails from West Sussex and now lives somewhere on the way to Neptune (though ordinary folk might say she lives in Northamptonshire). She enjoys writing short stories, supporting Arsenal FC – and spending her dad's money.*

# AN EXERCISE ROUTINE

## By Anon

I came across this exercise routine to build muscle strength in the arms and shoulders. It's suggested for the over 40's, but should work for all ages.

It seems so easy so I thought that I'd pass it on to some of my friends.

The article suggested doing it three days a week.

1. Begin by standing on a comfortable surface, where you have plenty of room at each side.

With a 2 kg potato bag in each hand, extend your arms straight out from your sides and hold them there as long as you can. Try to reach a full minute, and then relax.

2. Each day, you'll find that you can hold this position for just a bit longer.

After a couple of weeks, move up to 5 kg potato bags.

3. Then move up to 25 kg potato bags.

4. Eventually try to get to where you can lift a 50 kg potato bag in each hand and hold your arms straight for more than a full minute.

(I'm at this level.)

5. After you feel confident at that level, put a potato in each of the bags.

---

*About the author*
*This tried and tested exercise routine has been popular for many years. The editors would like to thank the original, unknown author for setting it down in writing and also Val for alerting us to its existence.*

# CURVE BALL

## By Elizabeth Bean (2006)

"It can't be possible; it just can't!" Jo whispered to herself as she looked down in disbelief at the little white plastic stick which had just mapped out her future. She picked up the instructions again, praying that she had somehow made a mistake. It appeared that she had done everything correctly. 99% accurate the box told her. Maybe she was one of the lucky ones? Yeah, fat chance of that.

This was the last thing she needed. A sinking sensation filled Jo's stomach, engulfing her with dread. Suddenly her legs felt weak and unsteady. She rested her forehead on the cool, white ceramic bathroom wall. "This cannot be happening," she muttered. But it was, and Jo's perfect life took a lurch into the unknown.

Yesterday, everything was absolutely normal. Jo was in love with Michael, they lived in a lovely cottage in the jagged hills of Halifax in Yorkshire and were due to get married the following year. She had just bagged herself a promotion from teacher to deputy head. Her work was diverse and challenging; something she really enjoyed.

Michael was sales manager for a large corporation selling office equipment, bringing in a good salary with handsome commissions. These paid for the twice annual holidays that Jo enjoyed so much, and for Michael's boy's toys.

The forthcoming wedding was to be an extravagant affair and was something that Jo had been planning, like most young girls, since she was twelve. She had the dress sorted: adorned with ivory silk and understated lace, fitted and uplifting around the bust and gently skimming the hips to end with a beautiful flowing train. It fitted perfectly (or rather would do when Jo got round to losing the half a stone that she had gained whilst on a rather boozy fortnight away with her betrothed a few weeks earlier).

Mental note, "Must re-join Weight Watchers." Scrap mental note… "No point now," thought Jo, smiling ironically.

Jo headed downstairs, grasping the banister firmly, concerned that her legs might give way. She absentmindedly picked up a cigarette (extra mild because they don't really count) and lit it. A moment of calm normality descended over her as she exhaled slowly, opened her eyes and observed the smoke's leisurely dance before it rose high into her own personal cloud. She took another drag before realising her actions, "No!" she cursed, as she stubbed the offender out.

Now what? What was she going to say to Michael? Oh heck, is it even his? No, it must be...it has to be! Oh heck, what am I going to do? Her brain was in hyper drive. When could this have happened? She knew she was late. Had known for a week or so but didn't quite want to admit it. Finally the burning desire to know, coupled with several sleepless nights and two million cigarettes later, she had bought the kit. It took her 2 days to pluck up the courage to urinate on the stick (how undignified) and now she knew. Unmistakably Pregnant.

It wasn't that Jo didn't want kids. But this would change everything. Of course the wedding would have to be postponed. There was no way she was waddling down the aisle like a duck. In any case the dress wouldn't fit and it was her dream dress; it simply couldn't be changed. Or maybe they should bring the wedding forward so that the baby was born in wedlock? Again, the same problem with the dress. She was too heavy for it as it was, and pregnancy wasn't going to make her any slimmer.

Her focus turned to Michael. How was he going to react? Would he understand? What if he suspected something? What if he thought she'd trapped him on purpose? "Oh, get a grip;" Jo told herself, "he was going to marry me anyway."

Her job; she had forgotten about that. She had worked so hard to get the promotion that she really couldn't let it go now. She suddenly felt overwhelmed and alone. She slumped to the floor and, drawing her knees up to her chest so that she could hug them, she rocked gently while a tear escaped, mixed with her mascara and left a dirty trail on her cheek. She wiped it away, with a mixture of anger and indignation.

Doesn't life have an amazing ability to throw a curve ball when you least expect it?

Jo was feeling a little calmer now. Shocked still, but calmer nonetheless. The real reason for her concern was a little indiscretion that she had had whilst holidaying with Michael six weeks earlier. Michael and Jo, despite being madly in love, were a particularly fiery pair when they disagreed on something.

One of their little altercations had happened in Tenerife, one of their favourite holiday destinations. They had hired a beautiful apartment in a gorgeous part of Los Cristianos.

On the day in question, Michael had decided to go on a golfing trip with a couple of men they had met the previous evening. Jo was livid, reminding him that they were supposed to be going on a boat trip that day. Michael flatly refused to buckle under Jo's pressure and told her that a day apart might actually do them good. This did not please Jo one little bit and there was a lot of shouting before Michael got up to go and attempted unsuccessfully to kiss Jo on the cheek.

"Great... don't mind me! In fact, I probably won't be here when you get back," screamed Jo at the already closed front door.

Jo stared, eyes full of tears, around the apartment. It took her a couple of moments of self pity before she dragged herself to her feet.

It was at that moment that she decided to go on the boat trip alone. She was a confident girl, she could make friends easily, so why the hell not?

Once the decision had been made, Jo glanced at the clock and, after a quick brush of her shoulder length blond hair, slid her sunglasses on and she was ready. She observed herself in the mirror. "Not bad," she decided. She had put a couple of pounds on but, thanks to her athletic build and her now healthy tan, she could carry it well.

Fifteen minutes later and she gingerly boarded the catamaran. The weather was fantastic. Clear ice blue skies, with just occasional swirls of high cloud, and around 30 degrees in the shade. Most of the passengers were in couples or groups of friends and, after a couple of bottles of complimentary beer, she began to relax and enjoy the feeling of the light sea spray on her body. She closed her eyes enjoying the sensation until she was abruptly awoken by a young and very attractive man. With a huge grin and laughing brown eyes he asked her if she fancied taking part in a champagne dive.

Jo was mildly embarrassed, partly because she had been snoozing and partly because the man was so incredibly good looking. She felt herself flush. "Oh, erm, no, I don't think so," Jo stuttered. The stranger was having none of it. He took her hand and dragged her to her feet. "Look," the guy said, "it really is lots of fun. I'm Carl by the way." Jo realised that her resistance was pointless and slipped her sarong begrudgingly from her hips. "OK," she mumbled in defeat.

Jo squealed in shock at the bracing water. It was freezing. "You'll warm up in a minute," Carl laughed, enjoying her discomfort. Jo heard the sound of people shouting on the catamaran before a large bottle of champagne whizzed past her ear with a spectacular plop, hardly disturbing the water. Within a heartbeat, all the men suddenly disappeared from view after the treasure. Suddenly Carl shot up beside her, bottle of champagne in hand, and a triumphant grin on his face. "Care to join me?" he questioned, looking at Jo.

Several glasses of champagne, countless bottles of beer and almost her daily allowance of cigarettes later and Jo was pretty drunk. She was enjoying the advances of Carl, and was flirting hard. She hadn't felt this good in ages. The trip had been wonderful. They had even been fortunate to see some dolphins which had swum gracefully next to the cat as if joining the race. Finally, the excursion was over. "Fancy a drink back at my place?" Carl enquired casually. Jo glanced at her watch. 6 p.m. Well, why not. "Love to?" she slurred.

Several hours later, Jo awoke, partly clothed, in Carl's bed. Her blood ran cold as she tried to remember exactly what had happened. Oh heck, she remembered kissing him....then what? She had absolutely no idea.

She glanced around the bedroom in the half moon light. Her watch said 10.30 p.m. She had a pounding headache. She had to get out of there immediately. She quickly gathered up her belongings before taking a final look at the gorgeous man, sleeping soundly on the bed, and let herself out of the apartment.

Jo's dishevelled appearance shocked Michael as she came stumbling through the door, some twenty minutes later. "Where have you been?" Michael shrieked.

"I went on that boat trip, and then went for a few beers with some of the crew," Jo explained. "I must have fallen asleep..." she offered lamely."

"OK..." he said. "Are you alright?" Jo nodded and rested her head on his chest as he wrapped his arms around her. That was where the conversation ended. The rest of the holiday continued without incident.

The phone rang loudly, startling her, breaking her concentration and snapping her back to reality. She eventually picked up the receiver, "Hello". There was no reply. She dialled 1471. It had been her mother. Glad she had not answered in time, she decided to ring her later after she had seen Michael.

Jo heard the key go in the lock, "Hi babe, I'm home," called Michael.

She took a deep breath, and replied, "Michael...there is something I need to tell you..." Michael walked through the door and put his suitcase down and hung his suit jacket on the banister.

Jo was about to object at his untidiness but thought better of it. "I did something really stupid on holiday," she said.

"What did you do?" Michael asked, concern showing in his face.

"You remember that boat trip I went on, the day that you played golf?"

"Yes."

"Well I met this really nice bloke called Carl, who looked after me all day. I got so drunk, that I went back to his apartment."

"And?"

Michael was taking this information extremely well, thought Jo, feeling unnerved. "And then I woke up in his bed, and I don't know what happened. And now I'm pregnant."

Michael looked at her before lifting her up and bursting into laughter.

"What is so funny? Did you not hear what I said? I have just told you that I spent time in another man's bed and now I'm pregnant!"

Michael gathered himself together, took Jo's hands and looked seriously at her bewildered face.

"The fact that you are pregnant is fantastic. It is quite possibly the best news I have ever heard. The fact that you think it's possibly Carl's is what is amusing me my love. You see, I played golf that day with Carl's partner. Carl is one hundred percent gay."

"What?" stuttered Jo, as suddenly everything clicked into place. "In that case, Michael, you are going to be a daddy."

"I can't wait."

"What about the wedding?" Jo asked. "I don't really want the baby born out of wedlock."

"Well, why don't we have a small ceremony now and then have a proper bells and whistles one after the baby has been born and you have lost all your wobbly bits?"

"Cheeky boy," she slapped him playfully. "But, yes, that sounds great."

And Jo's perfect life was perfect once more.

**About the author**

Elizabeth Bean wrote this short story in 2006 when she was off work with a relapse of symptoms. She hasn't had a formal diagnosis yet but is happily floating in "limboland", the place where many people with multiple sclerosis spend time prior to diagnosis, because symptoms mimic those of many other conditions.

Sadly, ill health saw an end to Elizabeth's ten year career as a sales consultant in the advertising industry. Wanting to keep her brain ticking over, she embarked on a creative writing course and has since written a number of articles for magazines. Her most recent venture has been a 75,000 word novel which she is hoping to get published in the near future. She is really enjoying writing and it is something that she wishes to pursue over the coming years.

Elizabeth has been married to her husband for eight years and they have two very lively boys: Matthew (6) and Daniel (3).

# I SEE DOT

## By Moira McDonald (2007)

I see my friend Dot's white hair from under my Dad's dark hairy arm holding the door open; there is no need for him to answer. I'm waiting for her to call for me; she is wearing her teddy bear dress.

We walk together to the railway sidings where the silver birch grows, Dad is going on his 12 hour shift at the steel works and warns me to clean the kitchen before Mum gets home from work; at the top of the tree I can see her walk down the path that crosses the reservoir in front of the house.

Our friend Sheila is waiting for us at the end of the road which leads to the sidings where the silver birch has managed to survive bombs that pock mark the unexplained spaces that we play in. Sheila is blonde, she is the same age, thinner though; I am dark haired and fat.

I help Mum to eat her toffee pudding, "Mum do you remember who I am?" She smiles, struggling to remember any words at all; "Why do I feel different?"

I hold Dad's hand whilst he is dying; he mouths, "Look after your mother."

The three of us climb the tree and look down the road.

I see my brother Stephen walking home.

---

**About the author**
*Moira McDonald, who was diagnosed with multiple sclerosis in 1995, is now retired. She has lived with her partner, Henry, for 20 years and has a son of 42.*

# A selection of poetry

# WILD COUNTRY LANE

## By Angus Alexander Brown (2001)

Sometimes I wander
I drift
As if lost in a land of dreams
Imagining that I breathe in
Sweet mountain air
Whilst wading through
Freshwater streams.

But the thing I like best
The thing I know for sure
Is that when I need to experience
The sounds of Nature close by
Of images both pure and serene –
When I need to feel safe and calm
To feel warm sunshine
A soft breeze or an April shower
I take a walk
Down a Wild Country Lane
By trees and fields
Of brown and green.

Away from all things artificial
Back to things deeper than just superficial
I venture forth to take an easy stroll
Maybe to stumble across a Woodland Sprite
An Elf or even a Troll –
Just to touch Magic
To smell the fragrant aromas
To feel the soil beneath my feet
To sit beneath an old oak tree
Or by an ancient hedgerow
To be **me**
To be **free**

This is my kind of Heaven
My Safe Haven
Just me and my favourite Wild Country Lane.

# AS DREAMS GO BY

## By Sally East (2006)

I hear the rasp of spade on sun-baked soil,
The scrape of metal on clay.
You are in your glass home,
Where plants as tall as men
Stretch their heads towards the sun.
Their ripening orbs turn from green to red.
How many this year?
      "Thirty nine, forty," you count

And with your leather fingers
You pluck the largest from its green umbilical cord,
A quick polish and into your mouth.
The juice bursts from its pulpy shell
And mixes with the sweetness of your lips,
A sweetness I know from your kisses.
Oh how I long for a kiss from that mouth,
As soft and syrupy as any berry.

Silver rain sparkles from the spout.
Geranium, sweet pea, lupin, foxglove:
The flowers that remind me of all our summers.
You stretch a strong arm
Above your hanging garden and tilt the can.
The tiny heads of blue and pink and purple
Tumble from baskets and nod
Grateful for the drink.

You stoop your aching back to tug
A dandelion from the earth
Before its golden head can turn to seed clocks

That spoil your carefully tended realm.
You stretch and wipe salty moisture from your brow.
Work done, you sink into a canvas chair.
The sun weighs heavy on your eyelids
And they close.

All is still but for a gentle wind
That ruffles your silver hair.
Are you sleeping, my love?
Shadows creep across the garden.
Blackbird sings his lullaby's overture.
Pigeon arrives for his supper of seeds.
The drowsy sun prepares to rest.
And still you do not stir.

I spy a butterfly upon your shoulder,
Wings folded. A silent movement
Reveals the colourful mosaic.
No artist's mind could conjure such beauty.
I watch it dance on the breeze.
Momentarily it rests upon
A slender rapier of grass
Beside the garden pond.

It then alights and rests
Atop the wooden sand tray,
Where memories of our grandchild's games
Are etched into the sandscape.
Then away, and to the shady arbour,
Thickly woven with honeysuckle, jasmine and rose.
It disappears from view
Amidst the foliage.

Beyond the hedge an ice cream van
Trundles by, humming a familiar melody.
It stirs you from your slumber.
Your eyelids part. I cannot see
The colour of your eyes from where I stand
But I know that they are blue:
Delphiniums are the same hue.
Mine are grey and pale in comparison.

Just as so oft repeated
In nature you are
The more handsome of us two:
A peacock to a hen.
I fill a glass with water and take it to you.
      "Did you sleep well?" I ask.
      "My dear," you say.
"I've had such dreams.

I dreamt first that I was looking out to sea,
Where white-sailed yachts were floating on the deep.
And then I dreamt that I was in the desert,
The golden sand stretched before me
Unto the horizon. Once more
I dreamt and this time I was in a jungle:
A tangle of lush vegetation
Smelling sweetly of nectar.

That is what I dreamt. And you? What have you done?"
      "I have seen a miracle," I say.
"The sea that you dreamt of is the garden pond
Where elderflower petals float like tiny sailing boats.
The desert is the sand tray. See where
Our grandchild's play has left a rippled, dunescape.
And lastly the jungle is the arbour.
The scent of honeysuckle and rose filled your dream."

      "You are wise, my love. I was dreaming
Of my own garden and yet through tiny eyes.
Our cottage garden seemed like
The whole world to me."
      "That is how it was.
You saw our garden
Through the eyes of your soul."
      "It seemed to me like paradise."

      "A garden can be paradise if tended well.
Your caring hand has made
A verdant world for us to share."
      "And now let's eat. Come Eve."
      "Come Adam, a meal I have prepared."
And arm in aged arm we stroll up to the cottage.
I glimpse a tiny movement and I turn.

A butterfly now rests where you were sat.

# POETS CORNER

## By Sally East (2006)

Wordsworth extolled daffodils
Dancing in the breeze,
Seamus wrote of peat bogs
And Housman spoke of trees.

Ted Hughes thought of foxes
Moving through the snow,
While Shakespeare's darling buds of May
Shook as the wind did blow.

Lewis Carroll made up words
Like 'brillig', 'slithy', 'toves',
And Robert Burns's loved one
Was like a red, red rose.

Who is the greatest craftsman
With lexicon and rhyme?
Too numerous to name them all –
You make up your mind.

# BIRD OF PARADISE

## By Sally East (2006)

'Neath canopy of paradise
Super troupers' shafts of light
Illuminate his terpsichore;
Erect he struts, the impresario
Gyrating on spindle shanks;
Needle thin and knock-kneed
He dances a samba
On stage of verdure;
Midst Elvis blue-black thrusts,
Steel rimmed amber orbs
Seek admiring and desirous glances

From the dour drab hen,
Mousy in her beige twin set
And mottled tweed skirt;
With nonchalant disinterest she exits
The arena; audition over.

**About the author**
*Sally East was born in Chadwell St Mary, Essex in 1965. Her keen interest in literature developed from an early age and she has enjoyed writing short stories, poems and articles, mostly of a humorous nature, to the present day. She is a member of Slough Writers and was delighted to be awarded 'Writer of the Year' in 2006. Sally has had some success in writing competitions. She is currently working on two novels – one in the romantic comedy genre and the other a children's story. Sally is a committed teacher of young children with physical disabilities: she is proud to make a difference to their lives by aiming for the stars.*

# SHADOW

## By Glenda Brown (2003)

There is a darkening shadow at my heels,
Pale weight, formless; where it falls, it crushes.
My mother hurls herself into its path –
selfless love and useless reason –
and my friends mouth prayers from a distant place.
The shadow falls, relentless, voiding all,
cast by a helpless one, powerless, numb.

# MEMO TO SELF

## By Glenda Brown (2003)

Light one last candle for me
while I wait for the stars to arrive.
Stars that will sing my name,
embrace my soul
and take me inside joy.
Tonight the world is heavy
and a little too long

so curl up my legs on the sofa
and gently move the cat,
don't think about tomorrow,
only light me one last candle
and place it in the window
while I wait for the stars to arrive.

---

**About the author**
*Glenda Brown has had multiple sclerosis for 13 years and was diagnosed with secondary progressive in 2003. She lives in West Yorkshire with her beloved husband, Tim, and cat, Miggy. Thanks to them, her mum, Jo, and her other unfailingly supportive family and friends, she says that she must now be one of the world's luckiest and happiest people and is currently working on both stories and poetry which explore these and related ideas.*

# TOUR DE ENGLAND

## By John Lake (2007)

Pumped full of steroids
Suffering from haemorrhoids.
You're supposed to be in France,
lost in Kent perchance?
Amazing! A Brit was leading,
'til nicked by the cops for speeding.

# WHERE ARE YOU?

## By John Lake (2007)

A man of the cloth atop his church spire.
What's that he's shouting may I politely enquire?
He questions his own life and belief
It's time God came down to give some relief.
Over two thousand years not a glimpse not a sign
For one of his own surely intervention divine?
'God where's that message you promised to send?'
'I've prayed 'til I'm blue, and I'm now round the bend.'
'How sick this world is so full of hate and sin.'
'How low must we sink until you see fit to drop in?'

The Vicar he died as his head hit the ground,
His God never showed, are you sure he's around?

# A SUMMER SONNET

## By John Lake (2007)

An English garden the perfect setting.
Manicured lawn blistered brown in the heat.
Customs maintained a Sabbath gathering,
this day every year the family meet.
Celebration in the summer sunshine,
white-shouldered children innocently play.
Mothers congregate quaffing dry white wine,
dads at the barbecue, cooks for one day.
Granddad recording, do something absurd,
uncle's playing football, red-faced not so spry,
youngsters scream and shout wanting to be heard,
toes dipped in water, auntie's skirt held high.
Rose reminiscences of times gone by,
until the day, like the sun fades and dies.

# M.S.

## By John Lake (2006)

Just two letters to change our lives.
Blissfully unaware, why should we care
for the anonymous thousands weeping Unseen?
Selfish hopes and desires,
that bike of Tebbit's had taken us far.

Her talent could move me to weep,
brushes and easel long since hidden.
Dark pain, numbed sensations, tears in her sleep.
Gentle waves breaking, slowly eroding,
impotent like Canute I cannot stop the tide.

Sweet smile and glistening brown eyes
that lift my soul and nourish my heart,
now rarely seen such sadness prevails

frustration and anger overriding all joy.
My love was chosen, why not me?

Our white-railed house no longer a home,
no knocks on the door, no cups of tea.
Old friends gradually faded and died,
a carer replacing a husband and friend,
stifled and trapped with no means of escape.

But hope will not abandon us forever.
Our children's innocent and carefree laughter
raise my love from her wheelchair and pain.
Each fleeting moment is beyond all measure,
a smile set free, proud eyes glisten again.

We measure no more by material gain.
Her gift has been stolen never to be replaced.
Yet many would swap their lives for our own,
for love lies content within our embrace:
we continue our journey two lovers as one.

# THE OLD RED LADY

## By John Lake (2006)

Streets turn to capillaries
feeding oxygen to the heart.
Seventy thousand cells bringing life into her soul,
she inhales deeply and stirs again.

Forged in history, unblemished by time,
Contemporary beauty enraptures all.
Once drawn in there is no release.
Infused, absorbed, lost in her embrace.
She takes everything but promises nothing.

Gorged, the lady can take no more;
the gathered throng, with but one love,
demand that she fulfils their need.
Able no longer to contain such power
her release brings such hope, such fear.

United! United! All shout as one,
Old Trafford is roused from her slumber again;
Echoes of thunder the world gazes with awe.
This woman of crimson and black:
Fulfiller of dreams, shatterer of hopes.


# EARTH, SEA AND SKY

## By Valerie Venables (2007)

### The Lie of the Land

The seismic shifts and tectonic plate drifts
of our shared lives have settled steadily;
no volcanoes erupt, nor giant waves drown
our vain hopes, and small dreams; we are becalmed
in the platitudes of the everyday.
Planet Earth, a suspended sphere in space
with no ropes or hawsers to anchor it.
String Theory might one day explain plainly
the globe's preposterous reality,
which now seems much less sensible than when
the earth was thought to be completely flat.
Heaven was above, and its four corners
filled with mythical beasts calmly grazing
in exalted valleys, gazing on peaks,
which pierced the clouds, and from whose sides bled down
the healing waters of mighty rivers.

### Sea Shanty

"The Sea, the Sea," is chanted out;
massed voices of the chorus shout,
in the voyager's "Sea Symphony".
I sing out too, a wild cacophony
with gulls and their screeches,
on deserted beaches.
And the sea and the sands are strands
of my lived life, while the wave bands
are tuned in to my internal radio,
as I listen to the tide's ebb and flow.

## Under a Blue Sky

Was above ever as bright and blue as this,
and the sun as glowing as new cleaned brass?
With birds fluting and thus strumming those strings
of the heart, whose rhythmical drumming sings
the low insistent notes of percussion.
I won't enter into any discussion;
I won't think of the sky and won't mention
the Doomsday image and the damage done
to the stratosphere, the ozone layer.
But how I wish that Pohjola's daughter
sitting on her colourful couch, the rainbow,
would weave a patch to fit, and then would sew
over the gaping hole and so repair
the catastrophe we have caused up there.

Author's note: This cycle of poems was written for one of the assignments in a module on Creative Writing as part of my degree course. The poems are all about me and how I live my life. The first one is actually about marriage (my husband and I have known each other for thirty years). Sometimes marriage can feel precarious, hence the imagery; things evolve differently than expected and viewpoints change, just as views have changed about the earth. My second poem is just about how I like to sing on lonely beaches. It features Ralph Vaughn Williams who based his "Sea Symphony" on Walt Whitman's poetry, which uses the analogy of a sea voyager to depict the course of a human soul through life (one of Whitman's lines became the title for a book and early film starring Bette Davis, "Now, Voyager"). My third poem concerns my worries about the damage humans are doing to the world. This poem was prompted by one of the few nice days of summer 2007 and the music of Sibelius. I suppose I should add that the first poem has hints of Handel. Music is one of my other interests, which I share with my husband.

---

### About the author
*Valerie Venables has been writing most of her life and has had a few pieces of her work published, mostly in magazines. She has recently had a carol published by Stainer & Bell in conjunction with The F.Pratt-Green Trust (The Carpenter's Carol, 2006). In 1994 she nearly had a book sold at the Frankfurt Book Fair! She has worked most of her life in nursing, mainly as a Health Visitor. She has somehow managed to also bring up three children. In retirement she is undertaking a degree in English Literature.*

# FERAL YOUTH

## By Joe Phelan (2007)

Feral youth – summer's day
piping hot,
striding down the bus,
slamming all the windows shut.
(I say nothing.)

Feral youth – pushing through
to stand triumphant
and head the queue.
(I say nothing.)

Feral youth – outside my gate,
shouting loud
spouting hate.
(I say nothing.)

Feral youth – against a wall;
a cowed young girl
giving all.
(I say nothing.)

Feral youth – tunnel vision.
Unaware of any schism.
My brother's keeper?
No, not I,
I keep my counsel
I do not pry.
(I say nothing.)

---

*About the author*
*Joe Phelan has worked in the racing industry for over twenty years but has always loved to write. He moved to the Isle of Wight some years ago and intends to commence a variety of writing projects including TV and radio scripts.*

# ALIASES
## By Marit Meredith (2006)

I wear many aliases,
added to, year after year.
Never complete
under any description,
but merely hiding behind more.
Not shedding,
but wrapping myself
in layer after layer.

# PREACHER/POACHER
## By Marit Meredith (2004, edited 2007)

I Remember
The local preacher;
otherwise known as
the Wise One, in tune
with the Earth, and with Him above.

Tickling trout, or
felling rabbits, swiftly.
One shot
to keep the population down
and put food on your table.

And for him? A living.
He was a gatherer, too,
of blackberries, blueberries,
mushrooms and bunches of
souls, in all their hues.

**About the author**

*Marit Meredith is Norwegian by birth and upbringing, but happily 'adopted' Welsh. Mother to six girls and grandmother to six (five boys and a girl), she returned to education as a mature student in 1994, securing an HND, a BA(hons) and a Postgraduate Diploma over the following few years, all within Art & Design and Art & Design Education.*

*Quite a bit of work followed, but ill health forced a re-think and she returned to writing, which has always been her first love. Marit has had articles, comments, readers' letters, a poem or two, a true life story and short stories published – and has several projects on the go – such as editing last year's nano-novel and preparing for this year's, editing and re-writing an almost forgotten manuscript (see the diary entries of the Would-Be-Protagonist: http://writelink.co.uk/blogs/mater), as well as working on a joint novel with her daughter.*

# TIDAL STRAND

## By Helen Clancy (2007)

The narrow sand bank widens
halfway across the tidal strand.
Insipid sea lies sleeping
on either side
of this thin
wrinkled causeway.
The ripples of the sand
are hard and lumpy
beneath my bare feet.
A path stretches out
as far as I can see
until it falls
over the edge
of the horizon.

All is calm,
no sign of life
no sound
except the breath
of the waves
in and out, in and out
against the furrowed sand.
I stand in silence
for just a moment
then I turn
and return
to our tiny croft
before the tide
buries my path.

---

**About the author**

*Helen Clancy is married, a mother of two children living in London. After studying English literature at A level and at Aberystwyth University, she is currently studying creative writing with the Open University. Her recent studies have re-kindled an interest in poetry. This poem is one of several that have been inspired by her love of the Outer Hebrides in Scotland, and of the ocean in general. This poem is not based on an exact location, but is an imaginary place, which is inspired by the stunning beaches of the Outer Hebrides, and could easily be a real place almost anywhere in the Outer Hebrides.*

# STORM DANCE

## By Athos Athanasiou (1998)

I find myself within a storm that's raging.
The rain is pounding down upon my soul.
The wind a gruesome war is waging
and on this coil begins to take its toll.

To show that to despair I am not ready,
I climb a hill amidst the howling storm
and there I see a rainbow strong and steady,
its power does to peace my heart transform.

This rainbow has a very different being,
it is not crafted from the sun's own warmth.
It takes a while to ken what I am seeing,
that from the moon its essence is brought forth.

I wonder how the moon can thus configure.
Perhaps this is not everything it seems,
for on the rainbow now I see a figure
a dancing and a twirling through the beams.

As it draws near I hear my heart beat pounding.
I feel the music through the dampened soil.
It starts off faint but then becomes resounding,
as if the very ground's about to boil.

And suddenly she's standing there before me,
bedecked in all the colours of that bow.
She smiles and takes my hand quite softly,
and dancing through the storm we start to go.

We tango through the forest,
do a jig upon the dale.
We break-dance in the bracken
and we shimmy in the vale.
We jive under the starlight,
and through the streams we bop
and though the storm still rages,
the dance we do not stop.

But now the moon lies still on the horizon.
The rainbow though still grand is growing dim.
I know that on the time she has her eyes on
and soon she must go back to join her kin.

She takes my hand and squeezes it quite gently
I try to thank but words are not enough
and though her exit's looming imminently
we smile for things are no longer as rough.

And all around me now there is a calmness.
An eye amidst the everlasting storm.
This eye will give me strength that I will harness
so that my dreams of peace will start to form.

**About the author**
*Athos Athanasiou lives in London and works as a software developer. He writes in his spare time, and has performed some of his poetry at the Poetry Café and at Farrago events in London. You can hear more of his poetry at www.myspace.com/athosfolk. He is currently writing a science fiction novel.*

# FLYING LESSONS

## By Kate Gooch (2006)

Today the air is full of teenage pilots –
As starlings, shrieking, screaming, learn to fly.
They land on twigs too thin, and perch, and wobble,
Their parents watching anxiously nearby.

I do not know a word of starling language,
Yet somehow hear exactly what is said;
Each squawk and fluttered gesture speaking volumes,
Translating into English in my head.

'Dar-ren! Come over here, now, with your sisters...'
'Mum! Mum! She's on MY twig, it isn't FAIR.'
'...Get off that effing pine tree, like I told you.'
'Mum! Dad said 'effing'!'  'Mike, no need to swear.'

'Dad! Dad! I'm hungry. Can I have a burger?'
'Get OFF that pine tree, Darren, double quick.'
'I'm flying! Look at me! I'm doing wheelies!'
'Oh, Mum – I think I'm going to be sick...'

'I'm bored, this flying's really, really boring –
Can't we do something else?'  'You're such a pain.'
'You're only saying that 'cause I fly better.'
'Dad! Darren's on the pine tree branch again!'

I close the door against the rain still falling
(This Spring's 'the wettest drought in history');
And leave the starlings to their lessons, grateful
The teenagers belong to them, not me.

*About the author*
*Kate Gooch is the editor of AVALON magazine, and regularly writes articles and poetry for various publications – sometimes under a pen-name.*

# UNINVITED VISITOR......

## By Sarah Roberts (2007)

Just who am I, since you came?
Will I ever be the same?
You crept up on me, slapped me on the back...
Wasn't invited, there's no turning back....

You try to take me over
Boss me all about
Didn't expect me to object...
Say NO! and scream and shout

You manipulate my senses
Turn my brain to fog
Shake me and pain me
Limbs heavy like a log

You came to change my life.....
Attack from deep within
But 'uninvited visitor'
You will never ever win!

*About the author*
*Sarah Roberts, who was diagnosed with secondary progressive multiple sclerosis in 2006, lives in London with her husband, Steve, and two daughters, Amy and Lucy. Sarah, having written this striking poem about MS, says that she now has the writing bug and will no doubt continue to put her thoughts down on paper.*

# SWANSEA BAY TIDE

## By Eiona Roberts (2007)

Serenely, so silently, the tide rolls in effortlessly,
So still, yet still rolling over this familiar shore.

A moment, a second, en-captures eternity,
The Spring tide brings hope for the future once more.


# CARPE DIEM

## By Eiona Roberts (2007)

I guess the concept was sound
If we'd but thought it all through,
But knowing me, knowing you,
We Carpe Diem'd

We took off for the coast
To the place we love most
But missed a vital signpost –
So Carpe Diem'd

We drove through mist and then fog,
Our wheels got stuck in a bog,
We looked at each other agog
But Carpe Diem'd

We sang songs passing time,
Oh such moments sublime!
But did we commit any crime?
No, just Carpe Diem'd

Ah but the fuzz when they came
Just had to apportion the blame
For setting the peat all aflame –
No more ...........Carpe Diems

# 9/11 – THE ORPHANS

## By Eiona Roberts (2006)

A peck on her cheek as he left for the station,
Not knowing the fate that awaited a nation,
A kiss gently blown to a babe not yet born;
A familiar scenario each USA dawn.

A stab through her heart when she heard of the horror
On CBS News, as she felt the world cower;
For death came so swiftly right out of that sky,
To husbands and fathers in the blink of an eye.

Today a child watches the world weep once again
As Westerners mourn for the day named 9/11.
Are pecks on the cheek and a kiss gently blown,
The only legacies left by fathers unknown?

Can each orphan resolve the grief of a nation?
Will they be the ones to lead Man to salvation?
For the powers that be took their freedom away
By denying all access to what happened that day.

Will the orphans of truth seek their own retribution
For atrocities cast against their own nation?
For Truth must be there, but knowledge is spurious;
Man, mourn this fact – the fat cat killed the curious.


# WHERE DO YOU GO?

## By Eiona Roberts (2005)

Where do you go
When your body deserts you,
When your mind is as active as ever it was?
To whom do you turn
When life overwhelms you,
But the cogs keep on turning
When they should be on pause?

Who bears the brunt
Of frustration and tears?
When your brain cells say "Yes",
But your body says "No!"?
To whom can you turn
When you're trapped in the prison
Of a body that's failing,
But your mind just won't go?

Who picks up the pieces
Strewn all around you
When your bits fall apart
Or no longer comply?
Who pays the price
For the anguish and sorrow
For questions you throw out
Knowing there's no real reply?

# MY CUCKOO CLOCK IS BROKEN

## By Eiona Roberts (2005)

My cuckoo clock is broken,
All he does is weakly shrug.
I must have wound him far too often
Or he may have caught a bug.

I really hope 'snot woodworm,
Or I must phone Rentokil.
Oh my poor old cuckoo
Let's hope you're not too ill?

Until I find what ails thee,
I'd have to stay in bed,
So I'm afraid my dearest cuckoo,
I've bought a digital clock instead!

**About the author**
Eiona Roberts lives in South Wales with her husband of 30 years. She is 52 years of age and has secondary progressive multiple sclerosis. Eiona has many hobbies including photography, swimming, poetry and music in all its forms, but mostly a love of the written word. She has already published a full length paperback book in February 2007 – 'Stumbling Along - A Journey with the Master of Surprises'. She continues to write but also volunteers as moderator of the Everyday Living Discussion Forums at the MS Society website www.mssociety.org.uk.

# MANIFESTING SUNSHINE

## By Irene Pizzie (2007)

When two cruel letters
struck,
and fear took hold,
I made a plan.

And so it began:

Magic Slippers
Many Signs
Marmite Sandwiches
Marks & Spencer

With each step forward:

Manifesting Sunshine
Miles per Second
Macaroons and Sausages

Unjust letters?
No – just letters:

Musical Symbols
Made in Switzerland
Mum's Silly

Maximum Smiles

# ONLY ONE SQUARE METRE

## By Richard Clancy (2007)

Fog covers the hills of stupefied Scotland,
bleak rolling countryside spoilt by an eerie foe.
Nowhere to see, no space to move-
the land, enveloped by a silent killer.

The desolate area, overcome as the fog descends
I stand outside, staring.
From a glorious countryside to a clammy, disorientating
nightmare-
I think to myself, why?
Why is this fog so dense, so consuming?
I ask the fog, it can't reply back, but instead it
just stares back, unable to find words.

I cannot find an answer.
I turn around, expecting at any moment to see a creature
of great monstrosity; I see none.
But what I do see, is claustrophobic, ghostly.
What I see, is nothing.
I put my hand before my face
and I see no hand.

I scream, but what is the use?
There is no-one here, except me.
I daren't move, lest I collide or lose my footing.
A fall here, could be fatal.
No wonder this fog seems murderous.
It wants me dead.
This is silly, I think. Silly.

I lie down, expecting at any time to be enveloped
by unconsciousness. I feel smothered,
stifled, scared, frightened once more-
as if I ever felt comforted!
It is getting to me, this fog.
I know I cannot break through
its impenetrability. I stand no chance; it is endless.

I might as well sit here and wait to die;
there is nothing else to be done.
I can see only one square metre.
As I lie there, in the middle of some Scottish countryside,
it is too much
I drift into inevitable sleep:
being able to see only one square metre is not enough.

*About the author*
*Richard Clancy is 14 years old and a student at Dulwich college in South West London. The poem was inspired by his love of the Scottish countryside, in particular the mountains, and also by his experience of the Scottish weather. Richard loves writing poetry, and creative writing in general, and hopes to publish more of his work in the future.*

# THE DOLPHIN POEM

## By Catherine Groffenberg (2003)

Dolphins have flippers
And swim in the sea
They make a sweet sound
And frolic so free

I love them so much
'Cause they are lovely to watch
As they dive and play
I never want them to swim away

*About the author*
*Catherine Groffenberg wrote this beautiful poem when she was 6 years old.*

# SWEPT AWAY (TSUNAMI 2004)

## By Sandy Lee-Guard (2005)

The day started well
Full of life, as known
Nothing unusual, just normal or so one thought
It was ...

Birds could be heard
A light breeze ruffled curtains at a window
Bed covers stirred
Voices began to be heard ...

A slight noise shattered the peace
It grew so quick
No time to think of what would happen
It was here – NOW!

This changed the course of life
For not so far away
A wall was rolling in
It swept away ...

---

*About the author*

*Sandy Lee-Guard, originally from New Zealand, spent the last years of her life in Slough, Berkshire. She was a dedicated and well-loved teacher of primary school children. Her other passion was writing and she has written numerous short stories and poems. A member of Slough Writers for the past two years, she was thrilled to have been voted 'Best New Writer 2007'.*

*Sandy's wonderful sense of humour and her Christian faith were often reflected in her stories and poetry.*

*Sadly, Sandy passed away in September 2007. She is greatly missed by her family, friends and pupils but her spirit and her writing live on.*

---

Editors' note: We are honoured to publish this moving poem and wish to thank Sandy's family and also her friend and fellow Slough Writer, Sally East, for making this possible.

# I AM THAT I AM

## By K.J. Howes (2007)

This is a story of words.
In this story one word follows another.
Each word has a meaning and each word has a feeling.

And the word is:

Wonder.
Joy. Beauty.
Love. Amazing. Best.
Innocent. Pure. Grace. Light.
Peace. Bliss. Enthusiasm. Playfulness.
Fun. Warmth. Gratitude. Enchantment. Delight.
Honour. Growth. Power. Divine. Abundant. Dreams.
Sacred. Heart. Blessed. Courageous. Happy. Strong.
Worthy. Excellent. Respect. Wise. Value. Intuitive.
Victorious. Good. Perfect. Successful. Brave.
Patient. Great. Spirit. Open.
Discipline. Humour. Winner.
Shining. Awareness. Health.
Me.
Myself and I

And you are the word.

And when you say the words, regular, you become the words.

Because you are it.

---

*About the author*
*Karalyne Howes, who was diagnosed with relapsing remitting multiple sclerosis in 2005, lives in Ashford with her cat Monkey Moo. Karalyne is currently working on various creative projects including running art classes for disadvantaged young adults, writing and working on a community performing arts project.*

# WHY SHOULD I FEEL HALF A WOMAN?

## By Julie Phelan (2007)

Why should I feel half a woman?
When I care just as much as a mother
when I yearn just the same as another
if I look at a new born child.

Why should I feel half a woman?
When I don't push a push-chair along;
when sleepless nights visit, helping prolong
the silence that keeps me awake.

Why should I feel half a woman?
When a Mother's Day goes by unnoticed;
when a child crying 'mama' sounds sweetest
when breaking my heart into two.

---

***About the author***
*Julie Phelan is a Learning Mentor for High School students and is also studying for a degree in English Literature to fulfil her desire to teach. She has had two short stories published this year and hopes one day to start a novel. She has been happily married for 18 years and her husband shares her literary and creative interests.*

---

# IF ONLY FOR A MOMENT

## By Sarah Daddy (2007)

If only for a moment
I wish I could remember
A minute without pain.
If only for a moment
I wish I could go back
To a life that hadn't changed.
If only for a moment
I would like to know
Why this had to be.

If only for a moment
To have the answer
Why this happened to me
My body just decided
With no option and no choice;
Provided no alternative
I didn't have a voice.
With every movement, every touch,
I am reminded of that day,
Reminded of a time and place
When I didn't have a say.
But, with each step, and day by day,
I find my outlook changing.
Days now passed, years gone by
With constant rearrangement,
I still have dreams and aspirations,
I'm still the same old me,
But, if only for a moment
I wish for how it used to be.


# FOR CALLUM

## By Sarah Daddy (2007)

I wonder what it would be like
To be your age again
To delight in every moment
Enjoy each time and frame
To see colour for the first time
Feel touch and hear sound
To taste, discover texture
And new smells all around
A tiny nose, those sparkling eyes
The laughter in your smile
Your first sneeze, your first word
The first time that you cried
You're such a special nephew
My happy thought, my joy
I can't believe you're one year old
My darling little boy!

# MEANINGS

## By Jan Porter (2004)

Sure of nothing –
I gaze deep, long.

Does the lily
know it's a lily?
Rare language of trees –
how does it flow?
Bud. Scent. Touch. Die?
How must I question?
What must I know?

Does the Whale
hunger dry worlds?
Soft shadow of snow?

The Tiger yearn blue ocean calm,
solid ships passing,
ghosting its sleep?

Does the Camel dream
forests, sparkling streams,
volcanic islands
ringed with fire?
Swaying higher –
touch rainbow peaks,
lost clouds?

Would the Blackbird forsake his garden?
Seek gateway of Heaven,
glory of Souls?

Sure of nothing –
before dawn steeples,
Truth unveiled
may tap at my door.

# ARTIST

## By Jan Porter (1998)

Pencil lines,
smudged charcoal;
the others sketch
and go –
taper like ghosts.

You conjure leaves like stars;
your crimson flowers,
golden spindrift butterflies
tremble with light
and fire.

You have known
monster caves where nothing grows,
circling hounds,
the blackest vertigo
paralysis of the soul.

You paint from Life –
green resurrection.

# PRINCESS

## By Jan Porter (2001)

She pines in the tower,
my sister, my shadow.
Trapped in ice chamber,
stares from the window –
mouthing the pane.

How can I free her?
Quick-silver her body?
Delve into the blackness,
Untie her tongue?
Can you cast spells?
Untie her fetters?
Dreaming, not living
too long behind mirrors,
my sister, my dear one.
Can you sing-song her?
From sadness, scatter starts –
make her believe in magic?

---

***The work of Jan Porter (by Elizabeth Porter-Cobb)***
*My sister, Jan, wrote the poem "Princess" for me when I was
diagnosed with multiple sclerosis in 2001, following five long
years of tests and horrible, surreal symptoms.*
*I was fortunate in chancing upon the kindness, support and
friendship of the Kent MS Therapy Centre in Canterbury. I wish
that all those who live with the torment of this dreadful disease
are able to find the sort of hope that I found there.*

# ME!

## By Shelagh Regan (2007)

When I sit among a crowd, I often feel the need to shout aloud,

Is it me! Or is it you! Can you see I am in pain, I am not vain?

But the ignorance you show is so very very plain, and drives me insane,

I am me! And yes I can see, and I am me! Yes I can feel,

Those of you who sit and stare and those of you who do not dare,

Please oh please why don't you try and see me as ME!

MS, what does it mean, it is not a bug, or something to shun.

We are like you, and you like us, so why is it we have to feel,

Like at the end of the long long sit, we are not like you, I am me,

I am in pain, I am not vain, but you could help to ease the day,

Light the way, and lift our day, and see me as you and as ME!

I am me! I cannot help the way I walk, or the way I talk.

You are thinking, I can see is she normal, no not like me.

I wish I was like you, but I accept I am not, I know I am me.

I try so hard to remember what you have said, but it's gone like a flash,

Why? Because I am me, and it's gone, but I'll bring it right back tomorrow,

You won't be there for me to show you, it is me; a new crowd is there,

As I am me! For new eyes to see, no they cannot feel the pain,

Or see me! No I am not vain, but help us oh please

Help us all with MS oh please I am like you but I am ME!

# THE BALLAD OF ZNORBARE

## By Heather Carter (1983)

Beware of the caves my pretty child
Be you timid or brave there are secrets too wild
For your ears.
There are legends too old to be whispered aloud.
Men stalwart and bold live in fear not too proud
To admit their fears.

Steer clear of the dark my adventurous son –
Be you up with the lark and when daylight is done,
Safe abed.
For The Creature still prowls far abroad through the night:
Hide your ears from his growls; hide your eyes from his might.
Hide your head.

'Tis said by the careless, the foolish, the drunk
That the creature is hairless, huge eared, with a trunk
And a tusk,
Crazed as a vampire hungry for blood,
Gasping out fire, foul breathed and you should
Stay in after dusk.

That monster is featured in fables, I know,
But was felled by The Creature with one terrible blow
From its paw
And the fear of the village still roams through the caves;
It's bloodshed and pillage, revenge that he craves
With his claw.

So spoke my father and his father before
The words and the warnings I chose to ignore.
With a head full of battles and brave deeds of yore
I went to explore.

My first faltering steps in the dark and the dank
Became bolder and braver as I entered the rank
Festering den of the beast – how it stank!
My heart sank.

Gone was the romance of battles of yore.
Gone was my image, a hero, what's more
From a curled up fat heap of moth-eaten fur
Came a snore!

The curse of my forebears, the scourge of the town
Slept on, unawares, all shaggy and brown,
Sublimely indifferent to fears and renown,
Head down.

A prod with the toe produced no reaction
But a snort and a grunt, a slight claw retraction,
So I drew back my boot and kicked him a fraction
To action.

With a roar, then a yawn, he stretched to full height
With bared teeth, unsheathed claws – then I saw that he might
Be ferocious. I turned tail and took flight
Into the night.

The bear in pursuit, talons raised for attack
I fled, and I stumbled to the floor in the black,
He came up behind me, his claw hit my back.
With a thwack.

My life passed before me as the sharp talon bit,
I waited for death, one last violent hit.
Impaling my back, he said – what a wit –
"You're it!"

---

**About the author**

*The Ballad of Znorbare was written by Heather when she was contemplating marriage. This contemplation was evidently fruitful, as Heather is married and has two daughters, two elderly cats and a lively dog called "Bryan".*

# A selection of memoirs

# IN SEARCH OF PADDINGTON

## By Gary Smith (2007)

I did it! Yes, I trekked to Machu Picchu, Peru in September 2007.

What an experience! Literally on top of the world!

First, a huge, heartfelt thank you to all the people who supported me and helped me raise £2,700 for the MS Trust. I truly could not have done it without you.

## A taste of my trip

Manchester to London Heathrow; Heathrow – New York; New York – Lima; Lima – Cusco.

Are we nearly there yet? After a day and a half travelling, we arrived in Cusco, Peru, to start our trek. Hadn't slept on the way over, didn't think I'd ever sleep again...but I would be proved wrong. A few days at altitude and I was off like a baby every night.

Meeting up at the Savoy in Cusco, we quickly found our feet, setting off on the 4-hour warm-up trek, and a taste of things to come. Savoy? What luxury. Actually, no – but it was clean and simple, just what you need to set you up for the experience of a lifetime.

Cusco was just the South American town that I'd imagined. Nothing like North American towns in the Wild West – these were "real" – and, as the Peruvians wearing ponchos and playing panpipes appeared from nowhere, it came to life.

"What's the weather gonna be like?" "Who knows," said one of our guides. "I just hope you've packed thermals as well as your swim-shorts..." I looked down at my bare legs...hoped I'd get a bit of a tan...

Clean, crisp mountain air was only the half of it. We experienced all weathers – from brilliant sunshine to golf ball sized hail stones. All of it against a background of some of the most stunning scenery in the world.

The people I met were great – all like-minded, determined to prove we could meet the challenge, trekking at altitudes of up to 4,500 metres. The air gets a little thin up there...but only one person had to withdraw, being brought down the mountain on a llama... somehow very dignified.

We sampled the local delicacy. Grilled guinea pig...tough, stringy, dry. Not something I'd try at home...and Christine would definitely have passed on that. The rest of our rations were more than acceptable. Lots of potatoes, vegetables, pasta, chicken. Better than I'd expected, to be honest...thought I'd come back a shadow of my former self...but in the event I came home only 2 waist sizes smaller – I put it down to the energy bars and snacks we ate mid-morning and mid-afternoon. Nothing to do with the Peruvian beer...

My wife had expected that I'd have at least one attack of the squits, and ensured that I had plenty of Diaralyte in my Medicine Pack. With the constitution of an ox, I am happy to report that I brought every sachet back home with me.

The camps were set up by the Sherpas, ready for our arrival each evening, and a warm meal already on the hob. How did they do that? Pack up after we left one camp and appear before us, ready at the next, for the night ahead? I think they'd done this before...

My boots were provided by Black's, and what a tremendous piece of equipment they were. I'd expected the biggest blisters in Peru – but not a single one appeared during the whole time. I wore them for about 3 months before I went, so they were well worn in. Nothing like the Sherpas' footwear... they seemed to prefer flip-flops.

My birthday fell 3 days into the trek. To my delight, the chef accompanying us very kindly provided a huge cake, with a slice for all 49 of us. What a surprise – never expected a party at 3,000 metres with a bunch of people I'd only just met, but par for the course: new experiences were around every corner.

Like when they left me in the loo as we arrived at the train station at Aguas Calientas. Happily, a friendly Argentinean we'd met told the group that I was still waiting for them...and it was only 50 minutes before I rejoined them.

And what a place. "Warm Springs" quite literally, very sophisticated though, with a swim-up bar located very conveniently at one end, with adequate seating all around.

Then Machu Picchu itself...how on earth did they do that? We were all quite stunned – and at the final destination of the trek. This was why we'd done it...and it was worth every single step, every single penny of fundraising, every raffle ticket, and every request for support.

The final farewell was a dinner in Cusco, when we reflected on our experiences. I unpacked the shirt that Christine had carefully folded and, amazingly, it looked fresh and crisp. Not like the rest of my gear, as I stuffed it away for one final time.

I returned home, exhausted but elated.

And Christine said, "Where do you fancy next then, I want you to do the Great Wall of China..."

I put my rucksack down... Got a bit of panpipe playing to do first...

---

**About the author**
*"Sherpa" Gary Smith could clearly give Indiana Jones a run for his money. Many thanks to his lovely wife, Christine, for writing up his adventures for us.*
*We look forward to hearing about Gary's next expedition. Spurred on by his wife's condition, he plans to do more treks to raise awareness and MORE CASH!*

---

# THE MYSTIC FERRET'S TALE

## By The Mystic Ferret (2007)

## Chapter 1

It was a dry day (unusually) when the doorbell rang and then rang again. I stood up to look out of the window to perhaps get a glimpse of who was there. It was then that my MS decided to play a trick on me! And I slumped to the floor, despite having a Zimmer frame in my grasp. As I called myself a few choice words, I realised something serious had happened.

# THE DANCER

## By George Church (2006)

She sways gently to and fro, as though suspended by a spider's silver thread, not threatening at all but simply graceful and her movements are beguiling, enticing and beckoning. Her glancing eyes call to me, persuading me. My face turns back reluctantly to the people who are speaking but I don't hear a word they're saying, not one syllable since I first saw the dancer. My peripheral vision catches her again and my eyes turn full on to gaze and admire, an emerald dress, flowing hair and long, long legs which step perfectly in time to the soft music. In the dimmed light at her best friend's party she is a shimmering bright silhouette against the anonymous grey dancers, entrancing, captivating and inviting. I brush past the other pale couples as I am drawn willingly, my hand outstretched, towards the beautiful emerald dancer.

She sways seemingly on fire, smouldering embers deep in her eyes, flickering shadows resembling tongues of flame and smoke leap across her form and the strobe lighting in the city club freezes her blazing figure in perfect stillness. On our first date the live music is stunningly loud with a heavy driving beat. Her flashing intuitive movements are hard for me to follow. She is so wonderful it's difficult to believe she is dancing with me. We have an invisible link preventing anyone else from breaking in. She faces me, a fabulous swirl of fiery movement, effortlessly burning in time with the drummer. We take a small break from dancing, ostensibly to quench the fire with a cool drink, and in a quiet lull she tells me.

She sways holding me close, dancing at the reception to a soft rhythm from the band. She moves with a motion like the molten gold of windblown forsythia, like a jewelled bead curtain recently touched, like a reed gently waving in a running brook. Dressed all in white she is as graceful as Tuesday's child. We were married that morning.

She sways with a gentle rocking motion, and our new son is soon fast asleep in her arms. She relaxes and settles back in the armchair, resting herself at last.

She sways and I move quickly to catch her before she falls but this time she's okay. We finish smiling and clutching each other. She knew when she told me years ago that her condition would deteriorate, perhaps with fortuitous periods of remission, but there would be a gradual and unrelenting decline. That's the terrible nature of multiple sclerosis. Laughing, her inept hands finally let go but for a few moments more I keep hold of her, my beautiful emerald dancer.

---

**About the author**
George Church was born in Birmingham and his childhood was spent in post-WW2 austerity (no TV, no computer games, etc.) and the playground for him and his friends was often the local canal. His wife Avril was diagnosed with multiple sclerosis in 1980. The couple now live in rural Wales with their son Andrew.

---

# The Mystic Ferret's Tale Chapter 2

Creative genius is like fog: you can see it but can you hold it in your hand? And so it is with my story.

As I lay there with a sense of foreboding (never seen her before?), it came to me that I must contact the outside world. My eyes (both of them) came to rest on the phone lying on the coffee table above me. It clicked into place that there was the very object I was seeking (it looked strange from this angle) and before you knew it, it was in my hand (and yet no one screamed) and then I dialled that most magic of numbers 999 and a soft voice entered my head, "Which service do you require?" Strangely, "All" went through my mind and the word "Ambulance" came out! The dog was looking at me from beyond the armchair, obviously trying to figure out this new game and how he should respond to it. It wasn't long before the doorbell rang again. "Déjà vu," I thought as my mouth uttered those immortal words: "Help! I'm in Here."

# THE FENCE PAINTING INCIDENT

## By Ralph "Salvador Dali" Edmunds (1997)

At the tender age of three, me and the girl next door, Elaine, hatched an idea ........ LET'S PAINT THE FENCE.

She was my senior by some seven days and therefore by accident of birth gets to shoulder the blame (even though the idea was mine and I provided the materials).

The brushes and paint were liberated from my Granddad's shed; the colour chosen was a beautiful white due to its wonderful contrast to the dirty, shabby untreated wood effect in place and the fact it was the only pot within my grasp.

Work began in strict adherence to union guidelines although it was never decided whose house was to be used for tea-breaks. Our inability to successfully complete such an onerous project of civil engineering left our Neo-rustic effect fence daubed with white gloss paint (influenced mainly by post-impressionism and Salvador Dali).

The sudden arrival of a near hysterical parent caused a premature halt to our masterpiece. She assured us, as she indicated the puddle of white gloss in which we sat, that the best method of painting was to put the paint on the fence not on the garden.

A suggestion of Action Painting cut no ice.

Next door but one stood Mr Winter, a sage-like spectator.

"Why didn't you call me?" pleaded Mum.

"They were enjoying themselves so much; I didn't like to stop them," the reply.

In later life I came to know that Mr and Mrs Winter were very keen music and art lovers.... Could this have been his real reason for not calling our Mums ????

Despite pleas from many of the world's great galleries, the need for a garden fence meant that this work remained in Leytonstone and tragically was never completed.

# THE PWDD AGM

## By Ralph Edmunds (2007)

I recently attended the AGM of the PWDD (Provisional Wing of Disabled Drivers).

There was a good deal of usual chat and people trading their stories. I was highly amused to hear Mike's story of when he went shopping with his disabled son:

A woman was parked in the disabled parking space. Mike kindly asked her to move and allow him to use the spot; the lady declined. At this, Mike left his car blocking hers and proceeded to get his son and his chair out of the car.

"You can't leave your car there!" said our caring friend, as Mike wheeled his son into the supermarket. "I'll be stuck here."

Somehow she didn't see the irony of the situation...

There was a good deal of discussion about what mothers say to their children as they park in disabled spots. Favourites were:

"Don't worry, they've got wheelchairs to save them walking..." or "Why shouldn't we be able to have the convenient parking space?" or "But I've bought too much to walk that far..." or "I don't want to spoil my new trainers..."

Have you ever noticed that when you are in a car park, people are quite happy to park in disabled spaces without having a blue badge but nobody parks in a spot that is marked "RESERVED FOR STAFF"?

As always there was a great deal of altercation between the members who think it OK for able bodied people to park in blue badge spaces (the sort who lend their badges to their relatives because it's just too much trouble to walk those few extra YARDS – they also haven't gone metric) and hardliners who want to let their tyres down and smash their headlights.

However there was some accord as two windscreen notices were approved:

"THANKS FOR TAKING MY PARKING BAY ..... YOU CAN HAVE MY DISABILITY TOO"

And a nifty Shakespearian note for use in posh areas:

"OUT, DAMNED SPOT! THOU HAST TAKEN MY SPACE"

But "WHERE'S YOUR BLUE BADGE YOU TWIT; I HOPE YOUR LEGS FALL OFF" was not approved, much to the chagrin of the hardliners.

---

**About the author**
*Ralph Edmunds, who is a member of the Kent MS Therapy Centre, has had multiple sclerosis for over 25 years. He now uses voice activated software to type and clearly retains his sense of humour, much to the delight of his friends and family. Rumour has it that he's devilishly handsome into the bargain.*

---

## The Mystic Ferret's Tale Chapter 3

In bounded the men in green, bows and quivers at the ready (nope! sorry, wrong image). For those of you worried about the dog it was fortunate that the wife returned from shopping to find a house full of chaos as the medics put their questions, to which I replied, "Right leg is at a funny angle (more than usual!)" and "I have a pain on right. $%$%& does it hurt." So in comes trolley (complete with g&t, NO!), but I did get the gas and air and once on that I couldn't give a %$%$.

# ANOTHER LAZY SUNDAY AFTERNOON

## By John Lake (2005)

*Come on Keano, put your foot in!* I shouted at my own private 28" football stadium. United were in cruise control again, seemingly oblivious to my exhortations. From my horizontal position on the settee I somehow managed the athletic task of reaching down for another can of the stress relieving nectar. God, I hated Sunday afternoons, thinking about the following five days' drudgery in a job I had loathed in its various guises since I started work 18 years ago. Today was worse than normal though because I had a course to go on; the thought of sitting around a table discussing the possible profit margins in brake pads was not exactly inspirational. I would also have to play the M25 lottery game to get there.

*Get in you beauty; about bleeding time.* At least we had 3 points in the bag thanks to another Andy Cole tap in.

Why wouldn't that knot in my stomach clear off and leave me alone? We were winning, I'd had a couple of beers, and it had been with me for so long that it even spoke to me. *Work tomorrow, you hate it, you deserve better but tough luck, don't worry though I'll be with you all the way.* With friends like that, who needs laxatives?

Debs got up to check the dinner; bang over she goes as if she's been shot.

"What's up? Has all that chocolate given you cramp?" My wife was stuck on the floor and couldn't get up. *Bleeding hell*, I thought to myself, w*hy does this kind of thing never happen when Corrie is on?* 15 minutes later and I've managed to help Debbie onto the settee. "Perhaps your legs are still drunk from last night," I joked, trying to reassure her.

Knock, knock; I can hear the arrival of an opportunity to get a couple of days off work. I phoned the man whose job title was higher up the ladder than mine (I don't have bosses!). *I'm really sorry, Paul, but Debs has had a fall and isn't going to be mobile for a couple of days. I know you must have paid out a lot of money for me to stay two nights in that one star bed and breakfast in Coventry, and I realise I could have changed the face of the car parts business industry forever, but it's out of my hands.*

Well that's what I meant to say but somehow it came out differently.

"Hello, Paul. I'm really sorry but Debs has had a fall and I won't be able to make the Coventry trip." Hey presto, a couple of days to sit at home and do nothing rather than have to go to work and do nothing.

Debs seemed to think the sensation would pass and told me not to worry. I couldn't sleep that night. Part of me was overjoyed at my ability to use Debs' accident for my own gain, but real concern was setting in about her condition, which had not improved. *Hello again* said my little gastric friend; *I've a feeling your real troubles are just beginning.*

**About the author**
*John Lake is 48 and has been lucky enough to be married to the long-suffering Debbie for 21 years; they have two lovely kids and live in Gillingham, Kent. John enjoys his writing, for which he's won prizes, and has previously had a story published. He became Debs' main carer in 2000 when multiple sclerosis began to affect her mobility and now he's working towards an Open University degree in his spare time. Underneath his cynical sarcastic cloak he claims to be a big softie.*

## The Mystic Ferret's Tale Chapter 4

Why is it that when you go for x-ray the pain relief seems to disappear, as the usual questions drift your way, "Please assume this position and hold!" which is a direct opposite to your normal function. It's a good job words are not shown on the x-ray as you mutter under your breath. After your brief introduction to yoga it all becomes a blur as it confirms your diagnosis and you are prepped for surgery. I do remember someone saying that I will be having a titanium hip, "Good!" I thought, "It will match the watch!" My time in the 'orthopaedics' ward was short lived as I became the victim of a chest infection which, with a low immune system, soon became rampant throughout my body at which time I was referred to Intensive Care (great fun).

# THE ULTIMATE ALPINE CHALLENGE

## By Mike Gallagher (2001)

It was certainly the most difficult mountain biking I have ever done and without question in the worst conditions, with the possible exception of cycling through a 40 mph sleet storm in Iceland.

For the Friday, a three-hour warm-up ride was planned to get used to the terrain and the altitude. We arrived in Morzine and put our bikes together in the blazing sunshine with the temperature at 26°C. A taste of things to come? I don't think so.

An hour into the ride we were feeling good, but the weather wasn't. Dark clouds gathered and within half an hour it was raining Alpine style; that's more like cows and sheep than cats and dogs. We cycled furiously to escape the appalling conditions that we weren't prepared for. When hailstones the size of marbles cut into our exposed flesh, I decided enough was enough and sought cover. The ventilation holes in my helmet were essential for summer riding, but I cursed them as they allowed the hailstones to burrow into my skull.

The next day, the challenge proper started – across the Alps to Switzerland and back again. Our guide announced, "The good news is that there is only one hill today." The bad news was that it was 6000ft high and would take between four and five hours to climb.

Half an hour into the ride, extra layers were being added to protect us from falling temperatures and the rain. The higher we went, the heavier the rain became, until eventually we finished up in the cloud itself. The rough and rocky terrain combined with the steepness put much of the route to the limit of my cycling ability. I was pleased that I managed to cycle it all apart from an impossible 100 yards. However, much of the steeper sections had to be done in short 100 metre bursts – more than that and my lungs simply gave out in the thinning air.

As the terrain became steeper, good mountain biking technique became more important. Too fast and you can't sustain it; too slow and you fall off. Not enough weight on the front wheel and it comes off the ground; too much weight on the front wheel and the back wheel loses its traction.

About five hours later I reached the top of the 6000ft hill. The reward for the pain suffered was the long downhill stretch. For many mountain bikers it is this downhill which makes the pain all worthwhile. In this case, a fast downhill stretch meant that our cold wet bodies would be chilled to yet new levels of hypothermia. As I careered down the other side, my eyes reassured me that my hands were on the brakes although I couldn't feel them. I thought of all that lovely, warm, winter gear I had left at home for this summer ride.

The route down to Chatel was wooded and afforded some welcome protection from the weather. It was a narrow rocky track with a precipitous drop on one side. The trick with highly technical paths like this is not going too slow – momentum needs to be maintained! Wishing to finish this challenge in one piece, I must admit to bottling out on some of the steeper sections.

Some of the fitter and younger types (approximately 95 percent of the group) clearly believed they were indestructible and attacked some of these highly technical slopes with gusto. More than a few demonstrated their ability to perform unplanned mid-air acrobatics without serious injury, although some of the blooded arms and legs did look quite impressive. As we descended into Chatel, the rain finally stopped and the sun came out.

With the biking finished, the queuing began. A queue to wash your bike, followed by a queue to get a shower, a queue to dry your clothes in the tumble dryer and a queue to get a beer. As we enjoyed a beer in the warmth of the late evening sun, we were optimistic about better weather conditions tomorrow; that is until our guide spoke. Apparently the snow line would be about 500ft lower tomorrow and, as we were climbing about 1000ft higher – we should be prepared for snow!

The next morning, I was wearing every item in my cycling wardrobe. The finishing touch was a plastic bag on each foot; my homemade substitute for my waterproof socks that were keeping very dry back in the UK.

After a couple of hours' climbing in torrential rain, we reached a mountain refuge offering coffees and hot chocolates. The attempts to dry out were fruitless and there was a distinct reluctance to venture back out into the inclement conditions. When we finally did, miraculously it had almost stopped raining. The clouds cleared, revealing a patchwork of green and white above. We zigzagged upward, crossing small snowfields with increasing frequency.

When we finally reached the pass at 7000ft, the sun actually shone, providing some spectacular views as the clouds jockeyed for position over the mountaintops. Within minutes, a huge bank of cloud swept up the valley, engulfing our ascent route somewhat faster than we had cycled it. We set off down the stony track into the valley the other side. Halfway down, the cloud caught up with us and our temporary respite from the torrential rain was over.

After reaching the valley bottom there was a long, steep climb to the next ridge before descending into Morzine. The meandering path, which was rapidly turning into a river, disappeared under the huge white snowfields at regular intervals. The steepness of these made it important to tackle them with care, especially whilst carrying a bike. (I had quickly established, after trying to cycle across one and making a rapid descent to the bottom, that walking was the only sensible option.) Some were so large it was a real challenge to find where the path reappeared.

Pushing more than cycling, we eventually reached the summit where we found a mountain refuge. It wasn't open in the height of summer, but we huddled between it and a large snow bank whilst we gave our flagging reserves a nutritional boost. The rain eased off momentarily and we caught another brief glimpse of the sun.

With the temperature close to zero, standing around at the top of a mountain when you are cold and wet is a good recipe for hypothermia; so after a rapid refuelling we were ready for the final descent into Morzine. The moment we started, so did the weather. The heavens opened once again, this time firing white bullets at us, which after a period gave way to torrential rain.

The muddy track down became more and more treacherous as the growing rivulets of water raced us down. Staying alive was the name of the game as we raced downhill at speeds of up to 30 mph. The intense concentration required to negotiate the continually changing terrain, mud, rocks, river, pebbles, gravel, etc., gave me quite a headache.

At the end of the fast and furious descent, it was questionable which needed hosing down more, the bike or the biker. After squeezing my brakes for half an hour, it was quite a challenge holding a hose.

Day four was the warm-down day. Again, I use the term 'warm' somewhat loosely! We actually started the ride in sun. Half an hour into the two-hour climb up the mountain the heavens opened once again. As if that wasn't bad enough I nearly got blown off my bike when a helicopter descended on top of me to pick up some equipment to take to the ski lift further up the mountain. The weather was so atrocious that the organisers decided to shorten the route.

We descended a narrow track through the woods, which had long since become a river. For half an hour I cycled down with my brakes full on to restrain the bike. When I got off at the bottom there was a sudden rush of blood to my fingers as my circulation recovered. A short run along the road took us to the finishing line.

On arrival, the Scope staff welcomed us by spraying us with bottles of bubbly. After getting off my bike and tasting some, I decided that the Scope staff had the right idea!

Editors' note: The 70 mad mountain bikers raised a total of £120,000 for Scope, thus helping to mobilise and give independence to a lot of people suffering from cerebral palsy.

---

**About the author**
*Mike Gallagher is a regular on adventurous fundraising trips, though he really is old enough to know better, and his lovely wife Sue puts up with his exploits remarkably well. "It all started 12 years ago when I climbed Kilimanjaro..." says Mike.*

## The Mystic Ferret's Tale Chapter 5

Well much of my transfer from the ward to Intensive Care is a haze, although some of my initiation to IC is a vague memory of needles and cannulas being inserted (no, not there) and smiling faces of nurses (or is it the morphine). A stack of liquid drugs plus food on my left and a stack of monitors on my right, to which this body was suspended in the middle on a form of bed, thank god for those ridiculous gowns even if they covered nothing. Oh and an oxygen mask on top of it all as I waited for the infection to consume me. Isolation bay and 24 hr nursing as I fought this bug.

# AND I HAVEN'T EVEN GOT IT

## By Hazel Lawlor (2000)

When Debbie, my daughter-in-law, contracted multiple sclerosis, we were all devastated.

Debbie and our son, John, had just become parents after waiting quite a long time.

I well remember John phoning with the news that he was to be a dad at last. Excitedly, I asked him how many weeks Debs was. "Not sure," he replied. "She's only just done the test!"

James arrived in due course to make them proud parents and making Bill and myself proud grandparents again after a gap of thirteen years.

Debbie seemed a little slow at getting back to normal but, hey, they had waited quite a long time for baby James; it was probably to be expected.

None of us knew that she was hiding something from us. Since the birth she had experienced pain and numbness in her legs and to some extent her hands and arms. She was a commercial artist and the loss of fine movement in her hands was a traumatic and terrifying experience for her.

She eventually sought medical advice and was told that, although tests were needed, it looked like multiple sclerosis.

John told us the bad news and that is when, to my everlasting shame, I can only say: I buried my head well and truly in the sand.

Debbie was far too vibrant a person to have something as dreadful as that. The doctors must be wrong.

I never spoke to her about IT; never asked her how she was, or how she was coping... I simply ignored it. I would ask John how she was doing and what was happening re treatment, etc., but I never asked Debs.

One day John said, "Why don't you ask Debbie yourself, mum? She needs to talk; everyone is ignoring it. Just talk to her."

Ashamed of myself, I went to the bookshop and bought a book on the subject I knew next to nothing about. I read it in one sitting and phoned Debs to tell her I was dropping in for a visit.

When I arrived, I asked her what she knew about the condition. "Not much, mum. They don't tell me much."

"Do you want to know?"

"Yes, I do."

I guess we talked for a couple of hours. I don't really remember. But after that things were a lot easier ... for me at least!

I had strange moments of irrationality, like when they gave her a Zimmer frame: I wanted to hurl it down the street. What was THAT THING doing in John and Debbie's house? (How I now wish she could swap the wheelchair for the Zimmer frame.)

Their family doctor was kind. He advised them that if they wanted another child not to waste too much time.

Along came Holly; James was four years old and loved his sister to bits. John and Debbie were certain they did not want James to be an only child.

I have often wished that I was as unselfish as Debs, but I'm not. I haven't got her big heart.

Eventually John gave up work to become sole carer for Debbie and the children. It was never easy and he has the scars to prove it. But after he suffered a total mental breakdown they at last got the help they deserved.

He was never cut out to be a house husband, but he has coped well and the children are short of nothing that love provides. He and Debs spend lots of time making sure the children have as normal a life as possible.

They both had great plans for the future, none of which included multiple sclerosis. Those plans are on hold for now, but miracles do sometimes happen.

John and Debbie have taught me a great deal. Debbie has shown me that whatever life throws at you, you can survive. John has made me proud: proud to be his mum.

The thing that Debbie, John, James and Holly have in abundance is love. Love for one another and I hope the knowledge of how much love is given to them by friends and family.

I have written this in the hope that it may give others the ability to communicate and not ignore any debilitating illness such as MS. You know what they say ... IT'S GOOD TO TALK.

A lot of love and a bit of understanding is all that it takes.

---

**About the author**
*Hazel Lawlor was born in Lancashire and now lives in Canterbury with her husband, Bill. She is mother-in-law to Debbie Lake, who has secondary progressive multiple sclerosis, a lovely husband and two delightful children. Hazel has had articles published in various magazines.*

---

# The Mystic Ferret's Tale Chapter 6

As I fought it with the help of staff and friends and family, some points stick in your mind despite the drug cloud, like the sister who constantly got my back up (boy! did we have a slanging match), a few choice words were spoken (only for me to find out, they were on purpose), did it make me fight!! And the ones who were there day and night just to perform a ritual (rock + roll) changing the bottom sheet, keeping me clean and tidy. Three times the family were called in as I lost the fight, only to hear the words, "He's back!" and even once as my stomach was being measured to the words of "54 Inches"; I've never been more than a 34" usually, just goes to show how infection can change you.

# COMBAT TECHNIQUES

## By Helen Birdsall (2007)

Well, Sunday offered a new dimension to this poxy illness.

There I was, peacefully carrying my dinner plate when the ground opened up and swallowed me whole (aka foot drop). Well out of the 3 of us, the wall did OK, not a scratch, the plate came off worse, ending up in the bin (complete with my Chinese takeaway grrr) and I came off somewhat a) embarrassed and b) cut! It was obviously a kamikaze plate that was happy to die for its cause but wanted to cause much injury on the way out. Therefore, it chose to embed itself in my left arm just above the elbow. All was not lost, however, as my bone stopped the plate from completely severing said arm!

So there I was, bleeding all over the place, hubby had had a drink so we had to call an ambulance, off to hospital, sirens and lights blaring cos I was bleeding so heavily – triage nurse took one look and through I went. 7 stitches, 8 butterfly stitches and lots of wine after (obviously), and poor hubby fretting like mad in a "hell, it could've gone in your neck or your chest and you'd be a gonna" kinda way.

Well, what I cannot get over and I'm sure it'll come in the end, but WHY doesn't my arm hurt??? OK, it's sore to touch where the stitches are, but considering it really did gouge a 2" deep, 1/2" wide cut down to the bone, I thought I'd be in agony... Not that I'm complaining, but do you think it will get sore or am I just lucky?

Editors' note: "Foot drop" or "dropped foot" is caused by reduced function in the nerves telling the front of the foot to lift when walking. Devices such as braces and splints, ankle foot orthoses such as Foot-up, Foot Flexr and the SAFO (silicone ankle foot orthosis), Musmate walking aids and functional electrical stimulators such as Odstock footdrop stimulators, Neurostep and WalkAide may reduce the number of trips and falls caused by foot drop, which is common amongst people with multiple sclerosis. Functional electrical stimulators must be fitted by specially trained experts to ensure that they work properly but are preferred by many users because they can help to improve residual muscle strength, whereas other solutions may contribute to muscle wastage.

---

**About the author**
*Helen Birdsall lives in the north of England and is a married lady with one 17 year old son (going on 7, going on 57). She has secondary progressive multiple sclerosis diagnosed in 2006 and now uses two crutches all of the time and a wheelchair when out or at work. Helen enjoys the usual range of pastimes from cooking (which she doesn't do so much of these days), pubs, cinema (though she always falls asleep), eating out (she's been known to sleep then too) and staying in watching TV with or without a Chinese takeaway.*

---

## The Mystic Ferret's Tale Chapter 7

It was about this time that a surgeon was called in at midnight'ish as my condition worsened again, and in my morphine dance I was asked if I would like to be operated on now or in the morning. For some reason I said "Morning"!

# EMOTIONAL FREEDOM TECHNIQUE

## By Irene Pizzie (2007)

I would like to share with you my introduction into the world of Emotional Freedom Technique or EFT, commonly known as 'tapping'.

Three years ago, I started experiencing some rather odd sensations in my left arm. For six months, I simply ignored it, until I mentioned to a friend that the episodes were happening more frequently, and that sometimes the tingling sensation led to weakness.

To cut a long (and I am sure familiar) story short, I saw my GP and was referred to a specialist. The tests began with an MRI scan, and continued with a lumbar puncture, blood tests, visually evoked potentials, and a further scan.

At the time of writing, I do not have a diagnosis.

At about the same time that I first visited my GP, I met up with a good friend of mine who had been studying a therapy called Emotional Freedom Technique (EFT). She helped me through a particularly emotional time using this technique, and I was hooked. It worked! A few months later, I went along to a course on EFT, and since then I have completed my practitioner training, culminating in becoming an Advanced Practitioner in January 2007.

During that time, I have had the pleasure of working with some wonderful people – and with myself.

*How EFT Has Helped Me*
At first, being sent to a specialist in neurology was alarming. I was convinced that a diagnosis of MS would follow, and that at that point I would probably want to die. Honestly. You see I had an overwhelming belief, and that belief was this: 'Diagnosis will make me ill.' (Do any of you recognise that one?)

Of course, this terribly negative and disempowering belief was not the only thought running around in my head. Oh no! There was loads of stuff in there; so much that I was floundering. I knew what depression felt like from an episode years before, and I felt I was back on the edge of the abyss.

Amongst other things I was running programs such as 'Having MS means I will die young'; 'I will be confined to a wheelchair if I have MS'; 'Nobody will ever love me if I have MS'; 'People that have MS are sad and depressed'; and probably worst of all 'Why me?'

When my EFT Practitioner friend first suggested a session to work on both the symptoms and those terrible beliefs, I was intrigued – but extremely sceptical. She explained what EFT was – that I would tap on various points on my face and upper body while saying some words. Hmmm, I thought, well obviously that will work! (I tend towards sarcasm if I am forced out of my comfort zone.)

Because this lady was a very good friend, and I was in such a mess that anything seemed worth a go, I agreed to a session.

*That First Session Changed My Life!*
Well you already know it did; otherwise why would I be sharing this with you?

Let me share a little of the background behind this wonderful therapy. EFT is a gentle, powerful, and empowering technique that has its roots in the work of American clinical psychologist Roger Callahan. Professor Callahan noticed that when a patient had a severe phobic reaction, they often had associated feelings in their bodies. He researched the meridian energy system, which is the system that acupuncture practitioners use when treating symptoms, and he started stimulating the appropriate areas for the reaction he was seeing.

Later, Callahan's technique was refined by Gary Craig (please see www.emofree.com for Gary's amazing website) into what EFT practitioners recognise today.

Rather than go in to the details of how to perform this process, I will simply encourage you to go to Gary's website and find out for yourself.

*So, How Does it Work?*
Imagine for a moment that tomorrow morning you are going to have to do something you don't want to do. It could be giving a talk, making a phone call, flying, anything that really scares you. Just for a moment, believe that this is really going to happen. I am sure you will have noticed that certain things in your body and your thoughts start to change. Perhaps you get butterflies, or your mouth goes dry. Perhaps you hear a voice that says 'Help!' Perhaps you see yourself getting anxious and not coping. The more you

associate with this imagined situation, the more your symptoms of fear are heightened.

How can this be? Quite simply, the negative emotions we experience manifest themselves as a disruption in our energy system. In fact, every negative emotion we have is a result of a disrupted energy system.

Simply tapping on a few meridian points, coupled with tuning in to your emotions, releases these feelings, and allows us to move on with our lives.

Since learning about EFT, I have tapped for all of my symptoms: my tingling arms, my numb toes, my intermittent lack of balance, the weakness in my legs. Over time, each of these has reduced. I now only experience the arm tingling about once a month; the other symptoms appear to have gone entirely. Remember, I am awaiting diagnosis, and I really am not making claims for a 'miracle cure' here! However, I should stress that persistence has been the key. I have made tapping a habit. I do it every day as a matter of course, and in addition use it at times of emotional crisis or anxiety.

*But Don't Just Take My Word For It*
There's lots of information out there about EFT, so check out the case studies on the www.emofree.com website. In particular, one entitled 'Dissolving MS symptoms with EFT – and a good look at the cause' is very interesting reading. You can find it at www.emofree.com/Multiple-sclerosis/multiple-sclerosis-symptoms-cacina.htm. Or have a look at the press release at www.emofree.com/Press-Releases/ms-eft.htm.

If you do an internet search for 'EFT, multiple sclerosis', you will find pages of ideas and resources, case studies, happy endings, and puzzling outcomes. But don't limit your search to one thing. As a practitioner, and believer in EFT, I 'try it on everything'.

If you do one thing after reading this article, please let it be that you type www.emofree.com into your browser and go looking.

You will be amazed, fascinated, and sceptical in equal measures. But hey, what on earth can tapping on a few meridian points do – certainly no harm. I dare you...try it!

*Where To Go Next*
If you are intrigued by EFT and want to learn more, you can find details of Practitioners and Training Courses at the Association for the Advancement of Meridian Energy Therapy website, www.aamet.org.

Carol Look, an EFT Master, has an exceptionally good site concentrating on attracting abundance into your life: see www.carollook.com.

And have I mentioned Gary Craig's website, www.emofree.com? By agreeing to receive the newsletter, which is filled with case studies on every subject, you can download the EFT Manual – which takes you through the process involved in tapping for anything you can imagine.

Happy tapping!

**About the author**
*Irene Pizzie BSc is an Advanced EFT Practitioner and can be contacted directly at freedom.foryou@yahoo.co.uk. She lives in South Cheshire with her four wonderful teenage children. Irene is a copy-editor, an Advanced Practitioner in Emotional Freedom Technique, and is studying to be a Personal Coach. Her dream is to awaken the world to the endless possibilities of creating abundance.*

# The Mystic Ferret's Tale Chapter 8

I don't think the surgeon was too pleased at being called out from home 20 miles away to hear me say that. It took several months before I managed to work out why I said that, and it seems that I figured it would be lighter in the morning so the surgeons could see better.

Anyway I was still alive when morning came and so was whisked away to be operated on, and apparently I stopped breathing for 20 minutes whilst on the table which my family were told (and I later found out). Coming round from the surgery in Intensive Care with a far more subtle painkiller, my mind could collate the past events and worked out that I seemed to be the loser in this battle with more losses than gains in the body stakes. How long I wondered before I would be stable enough to move into a normal ward and what it would be like to have the general public near and in the same ward.

# HELP!

## By Anthony Webster (2004)

### I may be a grumpy old celebrity – get me out of here!

I continue to take the Radio Times on a regular basis, mainly to convince myself that there's little worth watching on the television and therefore I can reasonably indulge myself throughout the evening with more worthwhile pastimes. Even from reading the listings, it is clear that the craze for makeover and/or celebrity programmes – and preferably the two together – continues apace. Celebrity cooking, dog-training, survival and quizzes have all had their turn, as well as through a celebrity's keyhole; the list seems endless.

Now I may have implied earlier a total disdain for 'the box', but in honesty it would take a major catastrophe for me to miss a rugby international – or the news several times a day.

It was the juxtaposition of these latter two one day a few years ago which led to a lapse in concentration and the discovery of, firstly, yet another celebrity programme and, secondly, the realisation that the word 'celebrity', along with various other words in the English language – such as 'wicked', 'cool' and 'random' – had changed their meaning while I wasn't looking, or listening.

The second of three rugby internationals had finished, the news followed and, before I'd regained my senses, another programme had started – 'The Alternative Boat Race'. With amazing speed and clarity, the 'voice over' explained the principle; 12 celebrities, 6 each educated at Oxford and

Cambridge, would vie for superiority along the Thames. The numbers worried me initially as I'd always believed that there were 8 oarsmen in each boat, plus the cox, of course, but this became a minor problem as we were introduced to the chosen 12. I only knew one of them – a disgraced politician – and I'd vaguely heard of a second, but I didn't know from where.

Had I dozed and woken several years later after all the celebrities of my own epoch had died off? This thought was quickly dispelled from my mind as my daughter's puppy passed through the room and she looked exactly as she had done the last time I'd remembered seeing her. The box was switched off whilst I re-gathered my thoughts. How could a person like me – one who keeps bang up-to-date with the news, reads widely from books, periodicals and newspapers, listens avidly to the radio – know less than 17% of a group of celebrities? Clearly the word had changed its meaning, as I mentioned earlier, but if that was the case, what could it now mean? Fortunately, as implied by the reference to the dog, one daughter was staying with me at the time so, after a quick rummage through the aforementioned Radio Times, and armed with celebrity names, I hailed her from the garden.

"Who's she? Have you heard of her?" I queried, pointing at a name below a photo.

"Isn't she the ex-wife of the former…oh, you know..." was all she proffered in reply. I didn't listen any further. A horrible truth had hit me. One could now become a celebrity by association – by association with someone who is, or has at some time been, famous.

"My goodness," I thought, "I'm a celebrity!"

Let me be brief: I've had a happy knack of meeting people who are, were or are going to be famous. As a young child, I shared equal billing (bottom billing as it happens) with a future Oscar winner and I went to school with the person who has probably written more film scores than any other living Englishman; no doubt he's got several Oscars as well. I've also played rugby against several (ex) international players, been to a Royal wedding and, whilst on the

Students' Union committee at university, worked alongside 2 future MPs and an NUS president who, as far as I'm aware, still holds a cabinet post. In my first teaching job, I was a neighbour of the second woman ever to be voted BBC Sports Personality of the Year and two of my former pupils are now BBC presenters. If I wasn't a celebrity under this new definition, then who was?

A great cloud hovered over me. After years of carefully managed anonymity, I was about to be grabbed by some frenetic TV producer calling me 'Darling' and all my incompetencies would be viewed by millions, in a studio kitchen, in a rowing boat, in the Australian outback or, worst of all, behind one of a semi-circle of modernistic lecterns, failing to answer questions proffered by a red-haired female dragon.

I would be belittled in front of celebrity taxi drivers and check-out attendants from Tesco who had served famous people at some time in their careers.

Thousands of former pupils would watch and realise that I'd only reached my exalted position as headteacher so that their education could be protected from my inadequacies. I would finally be seen as the weakest link.

My face fell, my brow furrowed and no doubt a whole host of other idiomatic expressions took over the rest of my body as the enormity of the horrors facing me sank in. I had become a veritable Victor Meldrew by the time my daughter re-entered the room – and it clearly showed.

"What's the matter with you, dad? You look like a grumpy old man," she opined as she passed through.

"Grumpy old man," I muttered as I grabbed the Radio Times once more. Leafing speedily through its pages, I found what I was looking for and read:

"Grumpy Old Men – 5 celebrities of a certain age complain about what is going wrong in our country and in the world at large."

**About the author**

*Tony Webster was born in Acomb, York. Having initially trained as an accountant, he re-trained and worked as a teacher from 1965, with some 'time off for good behaviour' in the 1970s to do research at Sheffield University. He holds degrees and diplomas at different levels from Manchester, Sheffield and the Open University.*

*Since his 'retirement' he has had several part-time jobs – some paid, some voluntary – including teaching English as a foreign language, proof-reading, youth work, church leadership and freelance writing for a BBC website. He currently holds a part-time position as post-graduate lecturer for a university.*

*His first attempt at writing fiction was published in 'York Tales', an anthology of short stories, in 2004. He has had short stories, poems and articles accepted for various magazines and newspapers.*

*He has been married to Gill since 1968 and they have three grown-up children and are also foster carers.*

## The Mystic Ferret's Tale Chapter 9

As I slowly regained my strength enough to face the public, I continually shared my apprehension of this to my doctors: "Will I be strong enough to fight off any infections around me?" To this my doctors replied that I would not move until strong enough, because they didn't want me straight back! (Make of that what you will.) Anyway they weren't sure as to where I should go, Orthopaedics or Respiratory, but in the end the latter won. And so as my bed was wheeled away from ICU to the strains of "Always Look on the Bright Side of Life" coming from my lips, I looked towards a new era and finally human companionship which had been sadly lacking. Now it gave a chance to escape from the soft food diet "which I looked forward to". At last real food and not something for 'Robocop'. Still had the trachea with the suction alert and was told, "Once that goes, then we shall see." Time passed by as I got used to a new routine and friends in a 6 bed bay. It's funny how you look forward to a bed bath! But in the back of your mind it's, "Has anyone got something that might put me back in ICU?"

# SOME DAYS

## By Deborah Lake (2007)

I was headhunted you know. Three quarters of the way through my graphic design/illustrator degree course a London design studio made me an offer I couldn't and didn't want to refuse.

This was back in 1985 and we didn't have the advantages of using Apple-Mac computers, which are standard issue these days. Everything from a c.d. cover to a glossy paged annual report for a major multinational company was planned out and created by my imagination and dexterity.

Now there are some days where I can't even write my own name.

I've got a sack full of badminton trophies. I was easily the best lady player at my club and there weren't many men who would take me on either. My boyfriend of the time (now my husband) was a pretty talented tennis player and eagerly awaited the opportunity to teach me a lesson on the court. He never won a single point.

Now there are some days where I can't bear to look at those trophies.

I used to love driving. I passed my test aged seventeen and still remember the sense of freedom that my first car, a little Hillman Imp, gave me. My boyfriend worked for British Leyland and he couldn't hold a candle to my prowess behind the wheel.

Now there are some days where my husband can't even transfer me from the wheelchair to the passenger seat.

After we married, my husband and I made the most of our free time. I was the major wage earner and a substantial part of our income was spent on holidays, sometimes three a year. Sun drenched lazy days on deserted Greek islands to week-long pub-crawls on the canals of England; we enjoyed life to the full.

Now there are some days where a simple trip to the town centre is too much to contemplate.

We've been married for over twenty years. My husband says I'm the best thing that has ever happened to him. He tells me that if it weren't for me his life would have been pointless and that he can't believe how lucky he was to meet me.

Now there are some days when I wonder why he stays with me, I feel such a burden.

My job took me to art galleries all over London. Evenings spent drinking champagne with the in-crowd whilst discussing the latest trends.

Now there are some days where I find myself looking forward to 'Emmerdale' or 'Deal or no deal'.

I'm lucky, or so some members of my family tell me. It could be a lot worse; at least I can still think for myself.

Now most days I'd love to swap places with them. Let them suffer the constant pain, the loss of pride and self-esteem, and the simple pleasure of just 'popping out'. Let them have to sit impotent downstairs unable to help their nine year old daughter pick her party clothes out or help their thirteen year old son prepare for his first date.

My husband adores me and vice versa; we do everything together. Since having to leave work we have become even closer. Our wonderful children have two parents at home to encourage them at school and to make the most of our free time. The friends we now have are reliable and true and we are making new ones every week.

Now every day I realise how lucky I am.

---

**About the author**
*Deborah Lake is 44 and now has secondary progressive multiple sclerosis, diagnosed in 1997. A former graphic designer, she is married to one of our editors and writers, John, who considers himself very fortunate indeed to have such a beautiful and intelligent wife.*

---

# GUILT

## By Lyn Kear (2007)

I recently went to visit some friends who live in Tiptree. They were very upset and exasperated by a local event. Two young boys aged only seven and eleven had broken into a local Special School and systematically, wielding hammers, destroyed all the contents.

If you knew me, you might be surprised to find that I could imagine the feeling these boys must have experienced as they carried out their exciting and daring plan of destruction. For I too have experienced that feeling of knowing what I was doing was wrong but having a greater feeling – backed by fear in my case – pushing me on to finish the deed.

The Primary School I attended, just after the war, was quite a rough and ready establishment in Widnes, Lancashire. The school building was a very large 'two decker' Victorian monstrosity with the Infants across the yard. The sexes were segregated, girls upstairs, boys below, but still the classes were large and my teacher in Standard 2, Mrs Murphy, ruled over a class of about 42 small girls. I say 'ruled' and she certainly did. She ruled with a rod of iron and a very sharp tongue. To be fair I don't remember ever being caned but the threat was always there.

We had annual exams and to me these were very important. I had a sister who had worked hard and passed the 11+. My parents were keen for me to emulate this achievement and Marjorie's successes hung over me like a cloud. Examinations were very important and we were tested and given a mark in every difficult subject from sums to story writing and poetry reading.

And yet handwriting was my worst nightmare.

We used dip in pens and that horrible ink that was made from powder and water. Our inkwells were often filled with blotting paper and if the pens were dropped the nibs crossed or bent. Well my pen nib had succumbed to the latter and as the exams came nearer my fears became worse. You must remember it was just after the war and there were not many luxuries about so my teacher only allowed us to have one pen nib each term. What could I do? I really needed to get a good mark for handwriting.

I spent sleepless nights worrying before I came up with my plan! I went over it in my mind until the fateful day dawned when I would carry it out. That morning I arrived at school early before many people were about. With sinking heart I crept into school and up two long flights of stone stairs. My heart was racing, my legs were shaking. I knew what I was doing was wrong. However, I could visualise my father's face and my teacher's sneer and, remarkably, fear drove me on. I approached the classroom door and breathed a sigh of relief because there was nobody in there. I expect the teachers were having a final cup of tea or a cigarette before they faced the day ahead.

The tall, heavy, painted wooden cupboard where I knew the nibs were kept stood in the corner beckoning to me. I slowly approached and heaved open the door. Fortunately I was very tall for my age so I was able to reach the shelf where the grey, cardboard boxes full of pen nibs lived. There were so many in one box alone and I remember there were several similar boxes lying side by side and we were only allowed to have one nib each! It hardly seemed fair. Quickly I opened a box and STOLE a new, golden nib and made a quick retreat the way I'd come and joined my friends in the play ground.

No one had missed me. No one knew what I had done and I don't think Mrs Murphy ever knew. I had got away with it!

Readers may be disappointed to think that nothing more serious appeared to happen after my act of grand theft. But now consider the age in which this terrible act took place – and that I remember the incident so clearly nearly sixty years after it happened. Of course I wasn't a 'Paragon of Virtue' as a child but then I wasn't usually naughty or daring either. I suppose there was a bit of excitement mixed in with the fear that drove me on, but I hate to think what my punishment would have been if I had been found out. I knew in my heart that I shouldn't have stolen but I am only human and a very real feeling drove me on that day back in 1952 – and I still feel guilty about that single pen nib to this day!

Editors' note: We have contacted Mrs Murphy who will be in touch with the author shortly regarding this most serious incident.

---

**About the author**
*Lyn Kear, was diagnosed with primary progressive multiple sclerosis in 1989. As a Primary School teacher, she continued working until 1990 when she took early retirement. She worked as head of PE in her school although umpiring a netball match was quite difficult.*

---

## The Mystic Ferret's Tale Chapter 10

Well it seems the revelations of the weekend (Chapter 9) will inevitably result in further chapters. Is that good news? Or what?!

# CAN YOU JUMP TANDEM?

## By Linda Holman (2007)

Way back in February 2007 I agreed to do a tandem parachute jump for the Kent Multiple Sclerosis Therapy Centre.

It was just by pure chance that one of the other members was talking about it and I made a chance remark that I would not mind doing one. Well before I knew it our Fund Raising Officer "Christine" heard and I had sponsor forms in my hand. The goal was at least £500. I did not think for a minute I would be able to do this, surprisingly I did. I did wonder what my family would think but they all said that if I thought I could do it then go ahead. They all said I must be mad.

I used the internet site www.justgiving.com. This made things easier as my eldest daughter told her work colleagues about it and they used it to donate. This way, after the jump, these donations were sent directly to the Therapy Centre and most were Gift Aided which meant the

Centre got even more. It was easy using the site and I would recommend it to anyone trying to raise money for charity. The way it works currently is that a small flat fee is deducted from donations made by debit card, and a percentage fee is deducted from donations by credit card, while the site handles all the administration, including Gift Aid.

The next tricky bit for me was getting my doctor to sign the consent form; at first he was not happy to do this. He wrote a letter stating his reservations but at the end said that he was sure I could do it. This was not enough and so I went to see him with the form and eventually he decided to sign it. Phew! I think that was possibly the most difficult bit.

Well for a while I slowed down on the fund raising as August seemed like ages away. Then suddenly July was upon us and I picked up my sponsor form and charged ahead with my fund raising. I was not the only one doing this; my mother who lives in sheltered housing was asking everybody in the building if they would sponsor me. She did very well and raised £89 for which I was very grateful.

My daughter's mother-in-law also was surging ahead with fund raising with all her contacts in her address book and others online. In the end the internet site raised £230 plus Gift Aid. Most of the people were leaving little comments saying either well done or you must be a nutter!

August the 5th arrived. We had the loan of the Thanet Multiple Sclerosis minibus. We arrived at the Centre for 9 a.m. for our journey to Weston on the Green. There were 3 of us doing the jump: myself, Dee and James (our driver). We loaded Dee into the bus in her electric wheelchair. It was a good job my husband (Peter) was with us. This was a learning curve because none of us had done this before and it was done by trial and error. Eventually everybody was aboard. Myself (Linda), Peter, Dee, James and, most importantly, Christine, who had been to Weston on the Green the year before so knew where to go and she had the paperwork. The journey was uneventful and we arrived at Weston on the Green.

All three of us had to go with Christine to register and fill in some more forms. We were told that we had a bit of a wait so all went back to bus. Meanwhile my daughter Nikki had arrived with Margaret (mother in law) and my grandson James.

It was a wonderful day weather wise as we had bright blue skies and a breeze. We watched all the trained people doing their jumps. It was a while and then one of the other jumpers that day came and spoke to us, telling us all about what would happen.

The time arrived when our tandem divers came to us to dress us in our flying suits and tell us what was expected of us. This was very good as it put our minds at rest as he explained what would happen should he pass out or worse. Apparently the parachute has a little computer in it that if we were going down too fast it would deploy the parachute.

Then the hats went on, horrible little things, not flattering at all. Whilst he was speaking to us I found out what colour the parachute was so that my ground crew would know which one was me.

During this talk I had some more supporters arrive from Swindon so I felt that I really had no choice but to go ahead with the jump. I never thought that I would not do it but, with all the support I had, I just had to do it.

Well we saw the aeroplane come down: it was time for us to go and get into the aeroplane, very difficult walking towards the plane, very strong draft from the propellers, made my walking stick virtually take off. It was a good job I was being supported by Peter and Gavin (my tandem diver). Finally we were all loaded into the plane and we took off. I was quite amazed that the door looked a bit like a bread bin with a roller lid. It was very hot in the plane. While we were climbing to the 13,000 feet we needed to jump from, Gavin attached himself to me. He showed me from his altimeter that we were there; about 6 or 7 professionals jumped and then it was me!

Gavin helped me to the door and then I was looking at the ground. He tapped me on the shoulder to tell me that we were about to go.

Whoosh and we were diving towards the ground; Gavin tapped my shoulder twice to tell me that I needed to put my arms out as you see on the television. This bit while we were freefalling was lovely I could not believe what I was doing, then another tap on the shoulder to tell me that he was deploying the parachute, at that time the webbing pulled me very tight, it was like doing an emergency stop in the car, you go from 120 mph to nothing in an instant.

Then Gavin asked if I would like to fly the parachute. I declined. I was very happy just to look around me. All too soon we were nearly down. When we were in sight of the ground I had to put my feet on top of his, the ground came and we landed, unfortunately my right leg gave out but there was plenty of help and a nice young man came and helped me up. Gavin turned round and gave me a kiss and I thanked him. We had to move out of the way as Dee and James were following us, Peter came across the grass with my stick and we walked across to all my supporters, my legs felt like jelly so I was leaning on a gate while Nikki went and fetched a chair for me to sit on. A little while sitting on the chair and I was able to walk back to minibus, albeit very slowly.

I was completely shattered. Margaret came to me with a bottle of champagne but I really did not want alcohol after this huge adrenaline rush I had already had. It was a lovely gesture but she said to take it home. It was time to go. We loaded Dee in her chair into the minibus and then we were on our way home. We had a little hiccup as James started going the wrong way on the motorway. I soon had my eyes closed and missed a huge chunk of the trip home.

We arrived back at the Centre and offloaded. Back home to our little dog Gem, who was pleased to see us and greeted us madly. I had time just to get a drink and then went to bed. Very happy and satisfied at having done something I thought I would never do.

The next day I was really tired, did not do anything. The next job was to get the sponsor money in. I was very pleased I did not have any trouble getting it. I raised £800 overall. Of course some Gift Aid to come on top of this so it was a job well done.

Next thing for me to strive for is a ride in a hot air balloon.

Just watch this space.

---

**About the author**
*Linda Holman is 53 years old and lives in Canterbury with her husband Peter. They have 3 children, 3 grandchildren and have celebrated their 33rd Wedding Anniversary. Linda was diagnosed with MS 9 years ago; her balance is affected and she has MS fatigue, but she's not giving in. She's still mobile and determined to stay that way.*

---

## The Mystic Ferret's Tale Chapter 11

Finally the time came for the removal of my trach, which meant improvement in my condition. Now I had to look forward to a nod that I could have real food at last, and when it came it was like the third coming (absolute bliss on the tongue), it is only when denied it that you appreciate something (texture), I knew now that my next move would not be long, it seems you cannot sit too long before the next challenge is thrust in front of you, and just after you have got the routine down to a fine art you begin to see the signs, more checks more often and the odd glance that has a word in it "transfer", till finally it's said: "Moving to Rehab Ward" and a shudder and tremor not from the MS goes through you, then the stubborn bit comes in, "Bring it on" is said quietly to yourself as you are detached and on the move.

# A POSITIVE DIAGNOSIS

## By David Johns (2007)

I remember first noticing symptoms in the March of 2000, when I was playing football and had to take a penalty. As I kicked it, the shot was very weak. I went to my doctor who referred me for tests. But I did nothing about it until something happened a year later.

This time there were two key events in my then stressful

---

life: I had just had a very bad bout of flu and I'd been studying for an MBA degree via distance learning whilst working full time. Never mind my legs, my hands were numb and I really thought I wouldn't be able to take my final exams. But the Open University was very helpful and offered me a script writer, though in the end I took the exam and wrote for myself. I passed.

Fortunately I had private medical insurance that enabled me to have an MRI scan and other tests which confirmed MS – and not a brain haemorrhage as first suspected. MS meant nothing to me. At that time I had no support and had to find out about MS myself. The neurologist who diagnosed me simply said, "You have MS and there is no cure"! The NHS at that time did not prescribe DMD's* and I thought my life was over. I felt so fatigued and drained all the time.

After diagnosis, I continued to work full time until I had the chance to take redundancy in December 2003. By that time, commuting was getting harder and harder. That said, I was still in reasonable shape and managed to get a new job straight away. Fearing for the unknown future, I used my redundancy to pay off my mortgage. The new job didn't pay as much but by then my focus in life had changed from having a successful career to my health and family.

Some years before, I had met a guy on a course who would change my life forever. David lived positively. His wife Steph was famous for curing herself of cancer through visualisation. I work in a very macho industry and, despite the stick he was getting from fellow course participants, David never once swerved from his positive beliefs. After my diagnosis I rang him and we spoke at length about refocusing my life's priorities.

Encouraged by David's outlook, I started to look around at alternative therapies. Eventually I went to the MS Therapy Centre at Letchworth (www.hertsmstherapy.org.uk) where I was able to have physio and reflexology, and the MS Action Therapy Centre at Walthamstow (www.msaction.org.uk) where I tried Reiki.

I really liked Reiki and decided I wanted to learn how to do it for myself. I found a wonderful Reiki master in my home town of Hertford who was prepared to teach me to Level 1. The attunement process I went through was very emotional and again helped me to adjust to life with MS. Jaqui was also a reflexologist and I decided to switch to her for treatment. (I have now also learnt Reiki Level 2 and one day I hope to be a Reiki Master.)

There are many aspects of my life that have been positively changed since I was diagnosed. But for my diagnosis, I doubt I would have met many of the people I have met. It has made me more relaxed in that I feel comfortable around disabled people and people of different cultures.

I follow the Swank diet for MS (www.swankdiet.com); take cod liver oil, a magnesium tablet, a vitamin B tablet and also a multivitamin one. Every day I do my stretches (from the MS Trust's exercise book), my stomach exercises for my core stability (taught to me by my physio at Hertford County Hospital), use a wobble board, either go on my exercise bike or go out on my bike – only bought a new bike a few weeks ago and found I could still ride it! I also do my Reiki daily. Once a month I have reflexology and also acupuncture. Trevor my acupuncturist has taught me to do self acupuncture 3 times a week.

With all these alternative therapies, I also take drugs as follows: Rebif 22 mg 3 times a week self injection; Modafinil for fatigue; Temazepam to help me sleep.

All of the above have been easy to build into my everyday life and are not time-consuming.

MS has not caused me to lose any friends; quite the opposite! I have made so many genuine positive friends since I have had MS that I actually feel I have taken control of my life and made it so much better for myself since diagnosis. And I still travel up to London to go drinking with my former work colleagues.

In fact, I feel so well and in many ways – not all, of course – feel better now than I did before I was diagnosed because of the positive life changes I have made.

There are a number of key people I must thank: David for teaching me the power of positivity, Jaqui for my attunement, teaching me Reiki and doing my reflexology, Trevor for teaching me self acupuncture (apparently my improvement due to self acupuncture has made me a case study in the world of acupuncture!) and finally my wife and children who have always been here for me, especially with the mood swings I suffered when first diagnosed. My wife was hard on me and made me do things when I could easily have let myself be a victim.

This is my story. I don't pretend I know the answer for everyone's MS but I do know one thing. If you remain positive and cut out all the negative people and influences from your life, your life with MS will be soo much better!

*Editors' note: DMD's = disease modifying drugs, also known as DMT's or disease modifying therapies, which are prescribed to some people with certain types of multiple sclerosis. Further information about current DMD's in the UK can be found at www.msdecisions.org.uk.

---

**About the author**
*David Johns was 41 when he wrote this piece. He was diagnosed with relapsing remitting multiple sclerosis in 2001 while he was working full time as a manager in a railway industry company; he continues to work full time in this highly stressful industry.*
*David holds an MBA degree from the Open University Business School for which he was studying at the time of his diagnosis – as well as working full time. He is a member of the Chartered Management Institute, Association of MBAs and also the Institution of Railway Operators.*
*He lives in Hertford with his wife Jan and his children Frances, Nadia and Davie.*

---

# The Mystic Ferret's Tale Chapter 12

Arrived in 'Rehab' with a flourish and a smile, thinking it had worked as got put in a bed by a window overlooking a courtyard. "This ain't bad," I said to myself, only 4 beds, but boy! Did I learn to regret saying that. The old MS mystery showed its ugly head when the old ignorance soon came knocking!! As I familiarised myself with my new surroundings something hit me, 'Radiator', right next to the bed!* And, as I found out, no way of turning it off!! HEAT!! Right next to me! Of all the things I didn't need. Immediately I rang my bell to summon assistance and by the blank expression I knew we were in for some fun! But that wasn't all it had in store for me as the days progressed. Why is it that a code exists for making beds when you don't need covers because of the heat, the number of times I have asked for them to be removed to a grimace of breaking the code! The next twist in the tale came one night as the window catch failed and a sound similar to the guillotine as the top window dropped 6" to send the curtains flying and a blast of icy north wind wake me! How many times I lost count. Only for the glass to crack on the last attempt. Only me!! Why me?!!

*Editors' note: Many people with MS are sensitive to heat, which can result in a most unpleasant worsening of function, which usually improves as temperatures return to normal. In fact, MS diagnosis used to be confirmed by subjecting patients to a hot bath: if their disability increased, they had MS.

# THIRD EYE

## By Charlie Crowther-Smith (2007)

I was 18, and working in my first job in the centre of Johannesburg. My route to work involved a bus journey to the central bus terminus, then a pleasant 10-minute walk to the bank in which I worked. The walk took me past a small pet shop and, being fond of all things soft and cuddly, I almost always stopped for a few minutes to watch the kittens and puppies as they frolicked in the cages that were strategically placed in the shop window so as to maximise their sales potential.

One evening in late December, the bank held a modest Christmas party for its staff – nothing too exciting, just a few drinks after work. Although I was, under South African law, old enough to drink, in that more innocent era I was unused to alcohol and was therefore rather feeling slightly woozy after the few beers I had drunk when I left the office for the walk back to the bus terminus.

However, I had my wits sufficiently about me to make my customary stop in front of the pet shop window. To my utter astonishment, the pet shop had gone, and in its place was a branch of a well-known gents' outfitters. My first thought was that I had somehow walked down a different street, or had stopped in front of the wrong shop – I was aware that I was not fully aware, so to speak, thanks to the drinks party. But a glance at the shops on either side of the outfitters showed that I was in the right place.

The more I stared, the more confused I became. I had stopped at the shop that very morning, and the window had been full of small animals. Now be-suited mannequins stared disdainfully at the passers-by, and rack upon rack of clothes filled the space within the shop that only a few hours previously had held cages, fish tanks, pet accessories and sacks of pet food.

Quite apart from my dismay at the disappearance of the pet shop, I simply couldn't believe that the change of usage had been effected so quickly, and with no warning whatsoever. Surely a number of steps should have been involved: firstly, notice that the pet shop was to close, then some sort of closing-down sale, followed by the emptying of the shop, its refurbishment as a clothes shop, and, finally, its replenishment with new stock and Grand Opening.

Bewildered, I eventually turned away and continued my journey home.

Next morning, feeling considerably better, I made my way to work, determined to resolve the mystery. I hurried to the shop, and stopped dead in disbelief. The mannequins in the windows had disappeared, together with the coats, suits, trousers, shirts, ties and so on that had filled the shop the evening before. Once again, the soulful eyes of puppies and kittens gazed up at me from the window.

I could make no sense of it whatsoever. For the next few days, I varied my route to and from work, just in case the outfitters I'd seen was actually in a street nearby, but there was no sign of it. Eventually, I decided that I'd imagined the whole episode, and put it out of my mind.

Then, about a month later, a "Closing Down Sale" notice appeared in the pet shop window. A couple of weeks later, the shop was stripped. A "To Let" sign went up, and the premises lay empty for a few more weeks. Eventually the sign was taken down, and shortly thereafter the shop fitters moved in. It didn't take long before I realised that the new tenants were...the same gents' outfitters I'd seen that night after the Christmas party.

---

**About the author**
*Charlie Crowther-Smith took early retirement in June 2006 from his job as a computer systems designer to become a full-time carer for his wife Fleur, who was diagnosed with primary progressive multiple sclerosis in 1995. Apart from his love of writing, and of tennis, which brought him and Fleur together in the first place, Charlie's passion is for amateur dramatics – if he won the lottery, he'd enrol in drama school the next day. "And I would leave you the day after!" says Fleur, who views all this "luvvy" stuff with horror!*

---

## The Mystic Ferret's Tale Chapter 13

The emergency team to deal with the window consisted of one man and several reels of tape, which of course were almost at their point of throwing away. "Still, it made a nice pattern on the glass," I observed. This was to hold it until the pane could be replaced, and as the days passed a reason had to be found for the inevitable "How did that happen!" I thought the explanation that I came up with was quite good: "It was from one of my high heels, as I practised for my part in 'The Rocky Horror Show'." It brought a few bemused looks, which helped as I was given a frame and asked to see how far I could walk, only to be asked to beat it the following day. If only I had known what I later found out after my discharge that I had 'C-Diff' and 18 people had died from the outbreak, and my emergency ileostomy saved me! And my later meeting with the Consultant Surgeon who operated on me who stated, "A normal person will take a year to recover from this, but, with your background, you can double that." I would have told them where to shove that frame! And the whinging on about trying to do it for yourself: "It's in your best

---

interests." Yeah!! "And my name is 'Attila the Hun'," I felt tumble from my lips!! Still the day came to replace the glass and what came next, "We have to remove the frame." With me right next to it! I can tell you I soon made a swift exit to the day room (a delight for all lobotomy patients) where I waited and struggled to retain my sanity. "Do I love hospitals," echoed in my mind.

# RELAPSE AND REMISSION

## By Ros Padgett (2007)

When I started my new job, it turned out to be just what I'd spent so long looking for. Little did I know that my life would be turned upside down just 18 months later when, in November 2000, my husband and I decided to take a few days away from it all. We went to our usual little retreat near the Norfolk coast to enjoy the friendly atmosphere and the welcome extended to us unfailingly by the locals.

This time was different. I started to feel a bit out of the ordinary after a few days, with numbness and tiredness and aching all down the right side of my body. I shrugged it off. After all, it wasn't the first time I'd felt this way and surely the break would do me good.

We decided to go for a little walk around the nearest market and then on to a nearby clothes outlet because I was absolutely certain that a bit of 'retail therapy' would take my mind off my ailments.

So there I was, on the point of buying the shoes of my dreams, when I suddenly came over hot, flustered and panicky. I couldn't help thinking, "I've got to get out of here or I'll faint." We went back to our B&B (with the shoes safely purchased) for me to have a lie down. After trying unsuccessfully to nap for half an hour, I still felt weird and decided that I needed to go home to get rest and sleep in my own bed.

We packed up, said our goodbyes and left for home. It was a familiar journey and yet this time I was a nervous and panicky passenger; all I wanted was to be back home. It was such a relief to get home finally. I'd never felt like this before. It was horribly frightening and I couldn't describe it to anyone.

After staying indoors for a day trying to ignore the numbness, I decided to drive over to my Dad's house for my usual Sunday visit. Except that I couldn't feel the bottom of my right foot on the pedals nor my right hand on the steering wheel, and I was getting more and more scared and feeling less and less safe. I made it a very short visit and didn't let on to Dad that there was anything wrong.

Unsurprisingly, I called work on the Monday and stayed at home to rest. But both my agitation and numbness increased and, after a doctor's home visit, I was signed off work for a week.

By the end of that week, I could walk only a few, unsteady paces and my GP came to see me. Three days later she started me on a long, tapering course of corticosteroids, which she felt would help my recovery even though I really didn't want to take them.

I'd been stuck indoors and off work for seven weeks by the time Christmas Day came. But I'd promised Dad that I'd spend the day with him and couldn't let him down. Although it brought back those by now familiar feelings of panic, my husband drove me over there. We had such a lovely time with Dad and some of the family that we ended up staying the night, with me promising to spend another couple of days on my own at Dad's during the holidays, which was a big step forward for me.

No sooner was Christmas over than I had my first of several visits from a physiotherapist. She taught me some invaluable lessons about walking, standing and balance. The very next day I was using only one crutch instead of two. This was definitely another 'step forward' for me. In fact, by the time New Year's Eve arrived, I was thinking "things can only get better" and threw a little party for Dad, who hadn't been well for a very long time and needed cheering up, and for my neighbours who'd been a tower of strength whenever I'd needed help.

A few weeks later I had an MRI scan at the Royal Free. This was my first hospital appointment since April 1997 and they told me there was a 75% probability that I had relapsing remitting multiple sclerosis. I understood it as "it may come and go" but I wasn't too worried because I'd only ever had bouts of numbness, etc., and it usually only lasted for a couple of weeks at a time. I'd always acted as if nothing was wrong with me and I tried not to let on to anyone else that I had MS.

About a month after being back at work part-time, I started to feel unwell and to get terrible panic attacks, so at that point decided to give up, get myself a little better and try to return again another time.

Then came another terrifying experience. I had a really bad reaction, including terrible shakes, to some medicine I'd been prescribed for anxiety. Rather predictably, a locum doctor was very quick with the command to stop taking it. But then I was faced with a month of increasing panic attacks, during which time I unwittingly slid into a deep depression that took me to the edge of a nervous breakdown.

Six months on and I went to stay with Dad for the weekend while my husband went away on a fishing trip to have a break from looking after me. By this time, I knew that I had agoraphobia and I hadn't seen Dad for a very long time. It was a shock to find just how ill he'd become and I lost a lot of sleep through worry that weekend. A couple of days later, Dad's condition became more serious and he was admitted to hospital. I got myself into a terrible state because I couldn't bring myself to leave the security of my home, even though I so desperately wanted to be with him.

My doctor prescribed me some medication for anxiety, but I still couldn't get myself out to be by Dad's side, not even when his condition worsened a few days later and the family were called to the hospital.

The following morning he died without me being there and I just cried and cried and kept saying to myself, "I should have been there." But the last conversation I had with Dad was one which I will never forget because I can hear him saying: "Just get yourself better and don't worry about me. I don't expect you to come and visit me; I know how you're feeling. Don't worry about me; just concentrate on getting yourself right and look after yourself."

I can't forgive myself for not going to see him, but when I think of how I was feeling he must have known what I was going through. Thinking back, we must both have had a premonition that it was to be our last weekend together, just the two of us together remembering all the good times we had, all the laughter. And that's exactly how I want to remember him.

My Dad was my rock, my world.

I was beside myself the next day. I wanted to wake up and find that it had all been a dream. I eventually plucked up enough courage to go to his funeral and sat outside the church with my mother-in-law. I couldn't go inside for the service but I knew he wouldn't have wanted me to get myself too distraught. That was the sort of kind and thoughtful man he was. Everyone understood why I couldn't go inside for the service.

But that day was to be a turning point. I decided that it would be the start of getting myself together, because I didn't want to let my Dad down. And I'd have to do it for myself; no one else could do it for me.

My mother-in-law asked if I wanted to go out for a drive the next day. I plucked up the courage to go and that was the start of not only getting out and about, but going out with someone else beside my husband. I also started walking outside and going a bit further each day.

I improved so much over the next couple of months that I astounded my husband by going out for a picnic with my mother-in-law on a lovely hot summer's day while he was away fishing. My confidence had grown so much by then that we all went out for a pub lunch the next day. That was the first time in a long while that I'd been surrounded by people without getting panicky. After that, I could feel myself getting more confident by the day, all thanks to my mother-in-law for getting me out.

Despite my protestations that I wasn't mad, my GP arranged for a psychiatric nurse to visit me. An earlier visit hadn't happened because of lost paperwork, but nevertheless this visit was useful because she helped me to build more confidence, handle more things on my own and aim for goals.

A year later and I had achieved a great many goals. I could go into a supermarket without panicking. I'd got a new car and gone a little way in it. I wasn't bothered by the two and a half hour drive to stay with my mother-in-law over the Christmas break. These were all achievements for me.

At my next hospital appointment, I wasn't in the slightest panicky and the consultant was pleased with my achievements. A lot of this was down to the nurse who'd taught me so much, and also the special equipment that Social Services had provided for me to use.

I persevered with driving throughout the bad weather and even went out to an evening social event with my husband, which was another milestone for me. As time went on, I gradually started to get the feeling back in my right foot and right hand and I found things improved for me as the weather got warmer and less damp. I noticed that I was tiring less and could go out to friends' houses and stay up a little later.

But my next adventure was a major breakthrough. We'd not been on holiday abroad for eight years and I'd booked a week in Rhodes! Despite worries that heat can affect people with MS really badly, the weather helped my MS and it was marvellous to feel the sun on my body. I didn't even need my walking stick as much as I did back home. So we decided to stay on for a second week and "forget about the extra expense if it's doing you some good" my husband said.

By then I could get myself in and out of the swimming pool and keep up with some of the pool exercises, splashing around even though I couldn't swim. I even managed to walk to the local village several times holding on to my husband's arm instead of using my stick, though we took frequent rest breaks.

Once back home, I got into the habit of using my stick only when out and not around the house. Everyone was amazed by this – and couldn't believe how much I'd done on holiday. After being back for a week, I walked down to the bottom of our road with my neighbour, having several little stops in between, and then to do some shopping in our local supermarket. It had been two years since I'd last done that.

The months have crept by with yet more improvements and I've achieved so much that I didn't think would have been possible.

I'll never forget what I went through and I doubt if anyone very close to me will ever forget. It's been a long, slow haul but worth the perseverance – and I have a lot to be grateful for and plenty of people to thank, especially my Dad.

---

***About the author***

*Ros Padgett has relapsing remitting multiple sclerosis and has dedicated this to her Dad, who was her rock. She is proud of her Dad for giving her the strength to deal with it and the encouragement to be as strong as him. She also says she owes her thanks to her husband, who had to work hard to come to terms with her MS but he has done just that, her mother-in-law for getting her to see that she had to help herself, her neighbours who have always been there when she's needed support, and all those who give up their time to help people like her with MS.*

---

## The Mystic Ferret's Tale Chapter 14

Editors' note: This chapter was written in June 2007 after powerful storms had lashed the British Isles.

Well after a long battle with frustration and getting nowhere, it took the power of 'Odin' to resolve my wireless router, OK! The lightning took out 2 tellies, video, dvd, aerial, phone, skybox, it brought me back online! And so the story continues as I return to my bed in the Rehab Unit, as I once more wait in dread for those fateful steps of the Physio and the long awaited words, "Shall we begin?" as a Zimmer frame is thrust under my nose (not literally) and the words, "Let's try a bit further today," like a cold chill down your back as you coerce the frame to do as it's told, "When's lunch?!" pops into your mind as a means of escape, when you know it takes your system 2-3 hours to manage the food, you begin to see nods of approval at your progress and the date of your expulsion is written down out of sight.

# YOU HAD TO BE THERE

## By Sue Crook (2007)

Look out Florida, look out Mickey Mouse; Sue was finally on her way, complete with iridescent walking sticks and family.

There was my son Stuart and his wife Sara with their children, Harry, Edward and George. A last minute edition to the expedition was Bradley, Sara's ten-year-old nephew, who really needed a break, as his mum had been ill for some time.

Unfortunately, Virgin Atlantic couldn't get him on the same flight or even to the same airport, so I volunteered to swap flights and travel with him. The trip was uneventful and the special assistance I required was surprisingly good at both ends.

We did have to wait two hours at Sanford airport while Stuart drove up from Orlando, but when he arrived beaming ear to ear my mood brightened immediately. He was desperate to show me the boys' toy he had been given to drive for the next fortnight.

It was a typically overstated and overlarge American people carrier, probably redesigned from a troop carrier. It really was very nice apart from the height of the threshold.

I suppose I should have thought more about making sure we were geared up for my mobility problems, but I imagined I'd do what I normally do and get by.

After a leg-up to get into said vehicle and a two-hour drive to Kissimmee we arrived at our non-adapted villa. (I know!) Two weeks and two flights of stairs up to my bedroom was a lot of climbing, and each trip out meant poor Stuart not only had to get my rented electric scooter in and out of the car but unfortunately I needed plenty of assistance as well.

My beautiful queen size bed really would have benefited from the presence of a fit young man to keep my feet warm. He would also have been extremely handy to pull the rope up that I needed to ascend to the giddy heights of my mattress.

I did get a little fed up when stuck in the bath whilst having a rest day, leaving everyone else to go out, especially as it was the only room in the house without a telly. (I told you, I know!)

Stuart, Sara and the kids packed as much as possible into the two weeks which was great but, with having to lug my scooter (and me) in and out of the car on top of everything else, Stuart did get a little fraught at times. The poor lad lost over a stone, most of it via steam from his ears.

The holiday was over and Bradley and I said our temporary farewells to the rest of the group, as again we were back to Sanford airport for the flight back.

A wheelchair was waiting for me but no staff; never mind, I managed to self-propel pretty well and when we took off I was tired but relaxed.

Half an hour into the flight and the Captain announced that there was a problem with engine number four, but not to worry. Why tell us then? A moment later he announced we were returning to Sanford as the engine had now caught fire. CAUGHT FIRE!

I couldn't remember what the stewardess had said to do in an emergency; all I remember was a lot of teeth and pointing. Where was my fireproof wheelchair and parachute?

We did make it back. As four hundred stressed and tired Brits invaded Arrivals, we made a damn fine job of spreading chaos and confusion throughout the airport.

Eventually the holiday rep announced that a hotel had been found capable of taking in such a large intake for one night, as our flight wouldn't be leaving until the following afternoon. I just hoped there was enough P.G. Tips to go round.

After another two-hour coach trip and a twenty-minute self-propel through the labyrinth of the hotel of the lost, Bradley and I collapsed in our non-adapted bedroom. (Not my fault this time!)

Two o'clock in the afternoon and we found ourselves on another coach returning to Sanford. What was that damp feeling? It's only water. Why was water lapping around my feet? Did the coach have a pool? Surely not.

Of course it didn't. Another wait ensued as we waited for the burst cooling system to be repaired. Never mind, at least we weren't on fire again.

I remember saying to Bradley that this couldn't be the end of our problems as we waited for yet another body search. Immigration control must literally know my body inside out by now.

It transpires that there was one more minor incident in store for us. The caterers had delivered the evening's à la carte meal, namely shepherds pie with instant mash and an olive on top, to the wrong plane; poor bleeders.

That was it really, back to England with no further incidents. I thought I saw a Gremlin sitting on the wing trying to rip an engine off, but I had been on the house red.

Three weeks after our return I did suffer an MS relapse. I'll leave it for you to decide whether it was a co-incidence.

**About the author**
*Sue Crook is 58 and not frightened to tell the world. She lives in Herne Bay, Kent and has two great sons, Stuart and Stephen, as well as 3 lovely grandchildren. Surprisingly she still enjoys travelling.*
*Sue has secondary progressive multiple sclerosis and was diagnosed 18 years ago. She did work as a carer for thirty years and always tries to remain positive. She is an active and most welcome member of the Kent MS Therapy Centre in Canterbury, Kent.*

# The Mystic Ferret's Tale Chapter 15

And so it comes as all things must to the end of my stay, when they say, "It's in your best interest" to get back into the normal world. Don't they get it!! It's normal where you are, you've become accustomed to the reveille at 06.00 hours and the 2 hour wait for refreshment and breakfast along with the daily 'Pub Quiz' of what to choose for meals that day, and the dissenting look when you ask for one of those rare things in hospitals (no, not doctors) a 'BIRO'!! When your day is mapped out like a military campaign and that squeaky chair beside your bed is being looked at with an ominous glance and you know the torture ahead, that once sat in you'll hear the words, "That's better, isn't it?" "YOU'RE not sitting in it!" jumps into your consciousness. Knowing that to touch the bed will bring down the wrath of above creates inner turmoil just as they do your daily checks (surprise! B.P. is high). And why is it that all is packed in the chair dressed ready to go at 8 a.m. and when do they collect you??!! Yes, late afternoon when everything has seized and bum stuck to seat and morale is at its lowest point, and they expect you to go out smiling ("pull the other one"). No fanfare! No balloons! No marching band! As one of their success stories is pushed out the door into a world of strangers.

Fini!

---

**About the author**
*Steve Whall, a master of suspense who is also known as the Mystic Ferret, is a popular figure on the MS Society's chat forums. His fellow chatterers were understandably worried about him during his hospital stay, but subsequently enjoyed reading about his adventures, which he serialised and published originally between February and August 2007.*

# IN PRAISE OF SPANISH HEALTHCARE

## By A.B. Dibble (2006)

I guess our first experience of Spanish healthcare came one very damp Christmas on the Costa del Sol about 12 years ago. Jan, my wife, had a bad case of cystitis and went to the pharmacy for some pills. She was given some Spanish pills of an unfamiliar brand. However, taking just one or two pills did the trick.

Jan then gave some to her mother when she also had cystitis. Again a couple of pills sorted out the problem. Another friend had an attack and one pill was enough. However the lady in question was rather worried and took my wife to one side. She asked if day-glow orange pee was a side effect. Jan put her mind at rest and apologised for not mentioning this earlier.

The pill's fame spread and soon no trip to Spain was complete without the purchase of a supply. One time we tried to buy a supply and the pharmacist said he only had a few of one strength left and offered us some stronger ones. Jan recognised these as the sort she had first been given. I asked her how the pharmacist knew to sell her the strongest and she replied, "Perhaps it was the way I was gripping the counter."

A few years back we acquired an apartment in Spain and the more frequent visits to Spain gave me ample scope to have further experiences with pharmacists and hospitals. Lamentably our command of the Spanish language is not great and each time we ask a pharmacist "habla inglais?" they always modestly reply "poco" (a little) and then prove to be fairly fluent in English.

Early this year I went to our apartment with a couple of friends. Both Jan and I suffer with the occasional cold-sore but this holiday I was quite unwell and had nasty cold-sores which I unwittingly spread across my nose and towards my eyes by the injudicious wearing of sunglasses. I'd always treated cold sores with Zovirax cream but with varying degrees of success so I went to the pharmacy and asked for Zovirax. "Doctors" I was told. Oh, I thought, I'll just wait 'til I get back to England.

We then passed another pharmacy so I thought I'd have another try. This time I was told "Doctor's, NOW". Well I can take a hint when it's put like that. I asked our neighbour, who although English is a permanent resident in Spain, for help and he took me straightaway to the smart new health centre where I was immediately enrolled as a patient by the English speaking receptionist and waited outside one of eight consulting rooms.

The lady doctor questioned me in broken English and gave my face, nose and eyes a very thorough examination. She prescribed a couple of things and said that there was a third which she may also prescribe if she could see me again at 8.30 the following morning. The doctor even made the appointment for me! I kept the appointment and whilst she was satisfied that the cold sores were not spreading she did give me the third prescription. In all I had a cream and two different sorts pills.

As I came through Customs on the way home, my face liberally daubed with cream, my friends said that I should put dabs of tippex on my passport photograph so that it would more closely resemble my face. We also joked about the possible lack of comprehensive testing by the Spanish drug companies. My friend suggested that the testing consisted of me letting the drug company know if the treatment worked.

Anyway, it turned out that one of the items prescribed was a supply of Zovirax pills which contained a drug called Aciclovar. This surprised me as I thought Zovirax only came as a cream. I didn't use the entire supply of pills, keeping some back for future use.

A few weeks later, feeling a cold sore coming on, Jan begged a couple of the pills from me. No cold sore appeared. Brilliant. For us this represents a miracle cure. Right, I thought, I'll try and get some on the NHS. I went to my doctor in the UK who readily gave me a prescription. Great, I'll try that again.

The next time I saw a different doctor who told me that he wasn't allowed to prescribe them despite knowing how hugely effective they were and then he proceeded to give me a lecture on the umpteen million pound savings he was required to make by the NHS. He said I could probably buy the pills privately and I asked how much they'd cost. He looked it up in his book and, rather embarrassed, said "They cost the NHS £4 for a pack of 25, h'mm that's not going to save many millions" and wrote me the prescription saying he could prescribe them no more than twice in a twelve month period. I took the prescription and thanked him kindly.

I collected the prescription from the chemist and ascertained from him that they would cost me £8 over the counter. So that's a 100% mark up for the chemist and even a profit to the NHS as, at £4, this is less than the prescription charge. To try and save money by not prescribing something on which the NHS makes a profit suggests someone's got their sums wrong. Either that or I've missed a basic point somewhere.

Either way it was a surreal experience which left me bemused. OK, I said to myself, let's try buying them privately as £8 is a very small price to pay to be free of cold sores. (Actually I've exercised my mind to try and put a figure on what I'd be prepared to pay to reach this blissful state and it's a tidy sum.)

Unfortunately this is the UK so it's not that easy. In order to buy them privately I still have to get a doctor's appointment and pay for a private prescription before the chemist will condescend to sell me some. S*d it, I thought, let's see how I get on in Spain.

The next time we went to the apartment I went to our local Pharmacy and asked for a packet of Aciclovar tablets. "No problem, that'll be 17.60 euros for a pack of 25." "Fine, I'll take two packets." At just under £13 for a pack this is probably less than buying it privately in the UK with no hanging around in doctor's waiting rooms. If I had bothered to obtain a prescription in Spain I would have got them cheaper. Yes, we now stockpile Aciclovar tablets.

More recently I had a nasty fall in a car park in Spain and the crowd that gathered round my crumpled form diagnosed a broken ankle. As our apartment is in a large expat area we have a spanking new hospital where the staff is multi-lingual and Jan drove me there. On the way, she took one hand off the steering wheel and reached over to touch my hand. "That's nice and caring," I thought. Then I realised she was checking for a pulse.

I guess that from that point on the treatment I received was about the same as if I'd attended an NHS hospital as, after I'd been assessed, there was quite a wait in the casualty department.

However I did spot an interesting notice on the wall of the casualty department. It told me that if I'd called a central phone number I'd have been directed to the nearest hospital with the shortest waiting time. What an innovation, a choice of hospitals.

I said before that the staff was multi-lingual. The porter pushing my wheelchair sang "Don't worry, be happy" to me and, when I joined in, laughingly said that I also knew the song. Fortunately a couple of x-rays showed that I hadn't broken anything but my leg was heavily strapped from knee to toe. I was given a prescription for Ibuprofen, a muscle relaxant but with possible side effects on the digestive system, and Omeprazole, a drug which eases digestive problems. I doubt that I'd have received a faster, better or more courteous treatment in England.

Incidentally, a neighbour of ours out in Spain snapped an Achilles tendon and was hospitalised for a few days. He was operated on very promptly and said the room he was given had nice views of the nearby lake and was like a private hospital in the UK.

So there you have it. A system where pharmacists are empowered to make basic diagnoses and dispense drugs. Drugs readily accessible and reasonably priced. Efficient medical care in modern facilities.

The next time we went to Spain I jokingly asked Jan which emergency service I'd use next. She said the dentist because if I did anymore stunts like that again she'd break some of my teeth!

---

**About the author**

*A.B. Dibble (known to his mates as Tony) was born of Northumbrian stock, as part of the post-war bulge. That's the Second World War for you youngsters out there. He says that he's lived too long in Woking and worked too long in insurance, a view unfortunately not shared by his boss who refuses to make him redundant or give him early retirement.*

*Tony is married to his third wife, Jan, who assures him that it's third time lucky. But he's only her second husband and he wonders if there's something she's not telling him.*

*Tony's plan is to retire to Spain as soon as possible to take advantage of the weather, cost of living and, probably, the wonderful healthcare system. His ultimate aim is to become a pile of sun-bleached bones outside a Spanish bar but he's envious of the recently deceased gentleman whose wife placed the following obituary in the Western Mail: "Sadly missed by his devoted wife and his beloved Sky Sports."*

---

# PASSAGE TO ENGLAND

## By Raja Varma (2004)

London (1952)

October 19, 1952. The P&O liner, R.M.S. Canton, docked at Tilbury at 11 a.m. Mr Bradshaw from the British Council had come on board to meet all the Colombo Plan scholars. He was a stockily built man from the north of England and not at all what I had imagined a British council employee to be. The people at the British Council in Calcutta where I used to go for their musical evenings as soon as my trip to the UK was confirmed were dressed in grey suits, unsmiling and very formal. Not a trace of emotion on their faces when listening to Beethoven's pastoral symphony, while my eyes were filling with tears.

Mr Bradshaw on the other hand, was dressed more casually and was very friendly. It turned out that far from being a high ranking official of the British Council, he was a minor employee and was formerly a courier at the British Embassy

---

in Rio. He asked me if somebody was meeting me in St. Pancras and gave me the address of a B&B hotel in Cartwright Gardens where I would be staying for the first night. "I will see you tomorrow morning," and with that Mr Bradshaw was gone.

The formalities did not take long (Mr Bradshaw had seen to that before he left) and we boarded the boat train to St. Pancras. The journey to London on that grey and dull October morning was depressing. The houses on either side of the track were grey to match the leaden skies; the trees in their back gardens, which backed on to the railway track, were leafless, and damp sheets, shirts, dresses and other items of intimate wear, were hung out to dry on lines like flags. England was not all like I had imagined it to be when, as a boy of ten standing on the veranda of my home in Mavelikara, I looked across the pond into the distance where I thought England would be; a bright, sunny place, with flowers, very similar to Mavelikara, but where the people wore different clothes and did different things.

But that first morning, on the train to London, I did not feel unduly depressed. It would be a new experience: I would be meeting interesting people, eating different foods; I would be a post-graduate student at London University; I would see Big Ben and Trafalgar Square, ride on the tube and on big double decker buses.

It was late afternoon as the train pulled into the sepulchral gloom of St. Pancras station. Baba, an old friend from Calcutta who had come to England earlier, was on the platform to meet me. "Let us go and get you settled into the hotel first. Tomorrow, we will look for a cheaper place."

The room in Cartwright Gardens, a crescent of Victorian buildings, was small, minimal and, to my horror, had no bath or toilet. The shared toilet was down the corridor. "Baba, how am I to have a bath in this place?" I asked. "There will be a bathroom where the toilet is, but you are better off using the wash hand basin in the room. You wanted to send your parents a letter to say you arrived safely?" We walked the short distance to Russell Square, and bought a couple of air letters. Baba was living somewhere in Earls Court which he said was on the underground line from Russell Square. "Let us have a sandwich and coffee at Platoni's bar and then I will take you back to Cartwright Gardens."

How well did I get to know Platoni's, which was to become the regular morning stop for a cup of coffee on the way from Russell Square tube station to the School (London School of Hygiene and Tropical Medicine)? By the 1970s, it had become a slightly upmarket Italian restaurant, although you could still have a coffee sitting on the high bar stool near the entrance. After Baba left, I lay propped up in bed (there was no chair in the room), and looked at the pamphlets given to me by the British Council. "The water from the taps is safe for drinking," one of them said. "When you are invited for a meal to an English home, always offer to wash up after the meal." "Do not clear your throat or spit in public. Do not burp; in India it may be a signal to your host that you have enjoyed your meal, but it is considered very rude in England." There were several other hints and suggestions in a similar vein.

My first night in England passed quietly. The view from the window in the morning was again of skeletal trees, but the sun was shining by the time Mr Bradshaw came to collect me. "They call it an Indian summer;" Mr Bradshaw said, "we don't usually see the sun this time of year." We walked across Russell Square with its leafless plane trees, through the University Senate house building and there it was, the London School of Hygiene and Tropical Medicine, where I was to spend the next three years.

"Ah, Mr Bradshaw, this must be Mr Varma," Mr Flatman, the head receptionist said. Mr Flatman was an ex-soldier; during his free time he could be seen shadow boxing and looked sheepish if he noticed that you were looking. "I will ask Mr Archard to telephone the Departmental Secretary to let her know that you are here. Professor Buxton is not in yet; he usually comes in at about 11." After talking to Mr Archard, Mr Flatman asked us to take the lift to the third floor. Walking along the corridor, we came across a door to the right. Not knowing whether to turn right or go straight on, we hesitated and were overtaken by a strange looking man in shorts and round steel rimmed spectacles. "I am

Professor Buxton. You must be Varma. I have to leave soon, but I will ask my secretary, Miss Wilson, to introduce you to Dr Bertram who will look after you."

Alison Wilson was a pretty young girl of about 20 (she was to celebrate her 21st birthday a few months later), with dark hair and green eyes; she wore a green dress matching her eyes. Over the years, I got to know her well and, when I was doing some field work in Ayrshire in the late 1960s, I visited her in Fairlie where she had moved following her marriage in 1955. Dr Bertram was a Scot and after I had seen him and gone through the formalities, it was time to go to the British Council in Davies Street. Mr Bradshaw took me up to see Miss Goodhart, a pleasant tall and thin woman with angular features, not at all like Alison Wilson. Miss Goodhart was the person assigned to look after me and two other Colombo Plan scholars who had travelled with me: Mr Razvi, a local government officer from Hyderabad, and Mr Mukerjee, a telephone engineer from Calcutta. Mr Mukerjee was leaving that day for Birmingham for his training.

After the British Council, Mr Bradshaw asked what I would like for lunch. "Have you had fish and chips before? No? It is typically English and you would like it." We went to the Lyons tea shop at the top of the Earls Court road and ordered fried cod and chips. I enjoyed it and when the waitress gave me the glass of milk I had ordered, I noticed it was cold and unsweetened. When I asked if I could have some sugar in it, she smiled and asked, "You a baby?" I could only smile back, but she did put sugar in the milk.

In the evening Baba came and took me and Mr Razvi to Earls Court. "I have got you both accommodations in a bed and breakfast place in West Cromwell Road. It is not far from Earls Court tube station. The couple who run the place are very nice." Mr Hendrickse, the landlord, was a cape coloured and used to be a sergeant in the South African police; a tall well built man, he was in striking contrast to his wife, a thin white woman with sharp features who looked perpetually harassed. Being a mixed couple in South Africa in the 1950s must have been a very unpleasant experience and would explain why they had come to England.

I shared the front bedroom with Mr Razvi. He had been in London before the war and had a degree from the London School of Economics, a fact which he would mention at every conceivable opportunity. "I must get an LSE scarf. If I remember right, there is a shop in Sicilian Avenue off Southampton Row run by Jack Hobbs, the cricketer. We will go and get one on Saturday." The shop in Sicilian Avenue was still there and they sold regimental and University and college ties and of course scarves. Mr Razvi bought the black, yellow and mauve LSE scarf and proudly wrapped it round his neck. "You see, Varma, now everybody will know that I have been to LSE (I wanted to tell him that anybody could buy the scarf, but didn't). I am wearing a Savile Row suit, but I can't open my jacket and show the label to everybody. This is much better."

---

**About the author**

*Dr Raja Varma was born in Mavelikara in the erstwhile princely state of Travancore, India in 1926. He was educated at the Madras Christian College, Madras, where he obtained a B.Sc (Hons) degree in Zoology in 1946. He was a Colombo Plan Research Fellow at the London School of Hygiene and Tropical Medicine, University of London where he obtained a Ph.D degree in 1955 and subsequently a D.Sc degree.*

*Returning to India as a senior staff member of the Virus Research Centre (now the National Institute of Virology) in Pune in 1956, he married Dawn in 1957 but, after she was flown back to England with polio in 1959, Raja returned to London in 1960 and joined the staff of the London School of Hygiene and Tropical Medicine, remaining there until he retired in 1991 as Professor of Medical Entomology. He is currently an Emeritus Professor of the University of London.*

*Raja now lives in Hertfordshire and has two children, Dilip and Dev. His hobbies include reading (biography and travel), visiting gardens, and enjoying wine and good food. This story and several others were written for his sons, particularly Dev who has primary progressive multiple sclerosis, and grandchildren Emily and Lucy.*

# MY TRIP TO OTTAWA

## By Michael Ogg (2007)

## Part I – The Dress Rehearsal

A few weeks ago I got an email inviting me to the retirement party of a good friend and former colleague at Carleton University, Ottawa. I'm sure nobody actually expected me to come, but that was extra incentive to try to get there. I still had some frequent flier points on Air Canada which operated direct flights from Laguardia airport in New York.

My friend Kathy came up with a brilliant plan: Carleton University has one of the best, if not the best facilities in Canada for disabled students, including fully accessible dorm rooms and 24 hour attendant care services. The facilities are available year-round. Kathy put me in touch with the right person and it was decided: I could stay there for 3 nights. I called Air Canada and was able to change my flights although there was only availability on the first flight of the morning.

But a few things had to go right. Firstly, I had to get to Laguardia. There are airport shuttle buses but only one carried wheelchairs and the times wouldn't work. New York taxis don't take wheelchairs. The only remaining option was to take the New York subway and bus. This needed a dress rehearsal.

I took the NJ Transit train at 9 a.m. and got to New York Penn station without a problem, as usual. But it then took me another hour to get to the E line subway because all the signed routes had steps and the elevators were out of service. This was why I was doing a dress rehearsal. Eventually I spotted a staff member pushing someone in a wheelchair so I tagged onto her and found the one working elevator to the platform. I finally reached a subway information booth.

The woman at the information booth was helpful, too helpful. She spent 40 minutes telling me things I'd already researched. Please, just let me onto the platform. It was the

New York wheelchair subway user's catch 22: you need a reduced fare transit card to open the special gate, but you can't get this card at the station. There's a form you have to fill out requiring a doctor's signature. Being in a wheelchair is not enough? "Before you get the subway, let me call ahead to make sure the elevator is working," she said. She called ahead: the elevator was working. I took the E line to Roosevelt Ave.

At Roosevelt Ave., I found the elevator. It was out of service. I pressed the emergency call button. It was also out of service. I couldn't get out of the subway but I couldn't even cross to the other platform to go back to Penn station. I waited for the next train and found the conductor. "I'll call the Transit Police," he said. The police didn't arrive. I found the conductor on the next train. "Go to the end of the platform and knock on the door. That's the subway operator's booth." The subway operator let me into his booth and called the Transit Police. When they didn't arrive, he called again. And again. And again. About an hour later, one policewoman arrived. "I can't do anything," she said. "I'm on my own."

There were a few stations with elevators further down the line but the operator said that they were all out of service. He then figured out the only way of getting me out: they'd put me on a local train which would go to the end of the line, turn round in a special loop, and finally bring me to the other platform from where I could take the express back to Penn station. The local train arrived but I couldn't get on: although the subway car is meant to be level with the platform, there was more than a 4" height difference which my wheelchair couldn't handle. I waited for the next train: same problem, but this time the operator and policewoman lifted up the front of my wheelchair and I was finally on the train. It took a long time to reach the end of the line and turn round, but now I was accompanied by an MTA staff who was instructed not to leave me until I was safe. We eventually got to the other platform; I changed trains, and got back to Penn station exhausted, hungry and thirsty. I took the NJ Transit back and arrived home after 5 p.m., tired and defeated.

## Part II – Getting There

It was Monday. I was meant to leave on Wednesday. I didn't know how I'd get to Laguardia. I called Air Canada and pleaded with the agent to work a miracle and get me on a later flight. Amazingly, he got me on the 16:05 from Laguardia arriving in Ottawa at 17:31. I was able to reserve the wheelchair shuttle from Penn station. I got to Penn station in good time and waited in 33°C heat for the shuttle. It didn't arrive, but at least I got a call on my mobile saying he'd be there in 20 minutes. After 20 minutes I called him back: another 20 minutes. Eventually it arrived and after more than an hour of New York traffic, I finally got to Laguardia.

The check-in agent was very helpful. He told me to find his colleague Maureen when I got through security. Maureen was equally helpful. She told me she was changing the gate to make it easier for me. There was a plasma display showing the weather. There were a lot of thunderstorms in the New York area. "The flight to Toronto is cancelled as the inbound plane cannot land at Laguardia." I wasn't worried: I was going to Ottawa. Then: "Flight AC719 to Toronto is also cancelled." Finally: "All flights to Toronto, Montreal, and Ottawa are cancelled." Shortly after, Maureen came to me. "There is a later flight to Ottawa," she said, "but we don't yet know if it will leave." "You can't leave me here," I said, and explained that I wasn't able to manage on my own. There was a flight about to leave for Montreal, the last Air Canada plane that had reached Laguardia. "Please try to get me on that plane," I pleaded. "If I can get to Montreal, we can figure things out from there." Incredibly, she got me on the Montreal flight.

In Montreal an Air Canada agent met me. I was back in my wheelchair and she accompanied me through immigration to the gate for the Ottawa flight. It was many years since I was last in Canada. I missed it: there's a calmness and gentleness that I don't find in the US. And there's bilingualism. Some extreme Québecois don't like the idea of anyone speaking English in Québec and some extreme Anglophones don't like the idea of a bilingual Canada. But I like it: there's a certain charm, quaintness, uniqueness. My

French is fairly good so I flipped from English to French and back. And yes, I did feel in a different country: maybe Paris on the St. Lawrence.

The continuing flight to Ottawa was short and uneventful. Again, an Air Canada agent met me in Ottawa. She wouldn't leave me until I was in the special wheelchair taxi, of which there were many. Fifteen minutes later I arrived at Carleton University. It was nearly 11 p.m.

## Part III – Ottawa

I asked the first person I saw how to get to reception. "Let me take you there." I checked in and was given the number to call for Attendant Services. I got to my room, called the number and a short while later Jaimie arrived. She explained how things worked and said that Alex would be along shortly to help me into bed and Scott would be along at about 6:30 the next morning. Alex used a free-standing Hoyer lift rather than the ceiling-mounted track lift that I use at home, but I've been lifted in a Hoyer many times before so was used to the routine.

Scott arrived at 6:30 and got me showered, using the shower commode chair, and dressed. He then took me over to breakfast. It was a fairly typical campus with dormitories that you'd find anywhere. But then I heard the bagpipes and a few moments later two columns of the Canadian ceremonial guard dressed in red jackets and black bear skin hats came marching towards us. The ceremonial guard is on Parliament Hill every summer. Its members are students from all over Canada who stay in the dorms at Carleton. It made perfect sense but was still a bit surreal.

At breakfast there was a wonderful sight: people in wheelchairs everywhere. As well as the resident students, many organizations bring disabled people to Ottawa and stay at Carleton University because the facilities are so good. After breakfast I went to the Physics Department and was overwhelmed for the whole day meeting friends and former colleagues whom I hadn't seen since I left Ottawa 13 years ago.

Richard's reception and retirement party was a truly wonderful event. It was so moving and emotional for everyone. Richard was dumbfounded that I'd appeared. The whole trip was worth it for that alone. But I hadn't come the furthest: Mette coming from Geneva had that honour. Many people said a few words, so I added some too. Richard had worked at Carleton for 30 years and he's one of those rare people for whom you can only say good things. I suppose we spent quite a lot of time together over the years: my research group had an apartment outside Geneva and Richard and I would often be there together. "You're going to do what?" he'd ask in incredulity as I headed off to a marathon cross country ski race in winter, or a day's cycling through the Alps in the summer. Like so many good friends and influences, I probably didn't recognize it at the time, but in retrospect the two most important people for me professionally were David at Cornell and Richard at Carleton. Thank you, Richard, for everything you did for me.

## Part IV – Trying to Get Home

My flight home was via Montreal. The plane was a fairly small regional jet so I had to be loaded with a special lift. In Montreal I had to wait quite a long time before the special lift arrived. I was getting worried because it was a tight connection. Eventually I was off the plane. A bit later my wheelchair arrived and I was lifted into it. I switched it on. Nothing. I tore into the baggage handler. "You've disconnected the battery!" Of course, this was a bit unfair because it was the Ottawa baggage handler who, quite unnecessarily, had disconnected the battery and not the Montreal one. But I was furious. "Without my chair, I can do nothing. Absolutely nothing. Do you understand?"

The flight attendant, the pilot, and the Air Canada agent conferred. "We're not going to make the connection," they said. "We'll have to put you in a hotel in Montreal" the agent said. "No can do," I answered. "I can't look after myself. I can't even transfer out of the wheelchair." "Is there anywhere you can stay?" she asked. I thought for a moment. Maybe I could get back into the residence in Ottawa. I called; it would be possible. She raced me over to the Ottawa flight. The same baggage handler who'd disconnected my battery in Ottawa met the flight, reconnected the battery and the chair worked again. I was so relieved it didn't even occur to me to be angry. Kathy met me and I took a cab back to Carleton.

## Part V – Finally Home

I was rebooked on the 14:10 direct flight to Laguardia. I had the whole morning so Kathy met me on campus on her bike. We went along the Rideau Canal to Hog's Back Falls. Ottawa's a fabulous city. Because it's the capital, special effort is taken to make it attractive.

I took a taxi back to the airport and eventually boarded my flight. I still had to get back from Laguardia, but we arrived in the middle of the afternoon so I knew that if all else failed I could take the bus. There was no point taking the Q33 bus because I knew that elevator to the subway wasn't working, so I took the M60 to 125th St. in Harlem. Plan A was to take the A line subway back to Penn station, plan B was to take the M4 bus. One of the two had to work. I got to the subway station; the elevator was in service. Yes! The subway was only 15 minutes back to Penn station and NJ Transit got me home a bit after 7 p.m.

There was just time to see Galen and give her the present I'd got. It was a native Canadian dream catcher necklace. According to native Canadian legend, the dream catcher catches bad dreams turning them into morning dew and lets the good dreams through. Someone had caught my bad dreams and just left me with good dreams.

*About the author*
*Michael Ogg has been entertaining Brits with his Transatlantic tales for a long time. But he's a Brit himself underneath it all. Despite rumours to the contrary, these binds into which he frequently gets himself really do happen and are not just staged for a good story. His next adventure will be to see how far he can get in Snowdonia.*

# SEE, LISTEN, REMEMBER

## By George Goodger (2007)

I worked for British Airways Baggage Facilities tracing lost bags worldwide. Also we held Lost Property that passengers had left on aircraft.

I remember once getting a call from Lady Powell, the widow of Baden Powell, the Boy Scout leader. She wanted the return of some Lost Property she had left at Terminal 2. We got chatting and she invited me to her Grace and Favour flat in Hampton Court. This was some years ago now and I wobbled a lot owing to my MS, so was taken by a friend of mine, Richard.

We parked the car in the grounds of Hampton Court and climbed the long, thin, winding staircase to her front door. When she opened the door it was like stepping back 100 years. Everything was antique: carpets, curtains and the décor. It was clean and dark in colour, but also seemed aged. The accompanying musty smell had you in no doubt it was all genuine.

Lady Powell was a typical lovely old person with white hair and bent over. We talked for about two hours and the experiences she told us about were so interesting; well worth the climb to her flat.

During my time with BA, I dealt with many celebrities from Cliff Richard to Dame Edna Everage, but one who sticks in my mind more than any is Muhammad Ali. He started sparring with me while I was filling out a missing report; he was lucky I didn't get angry. So you could say I fought The Greatest World Champion ever; he is a great man.

It enthrals me, meeting people with experience of life. Like my Dad, with whom I very often had conversations about his early years and war experiences. I feel sorry for people, especially the young, who will not listen; so much can be learned.

My Dad's tales of Covent Garden and knowledge of Musicals always fascinated me. His war stories I found amazing and I still cannot comprehend the enormity of how they could land on Anzio (in Italy) during World War II and be pinned down on the beaches for months under German gunfire. What men these people were; their sacrifice is something we should never forget.

In his own eminent phraseology he always ended by saying how he won the war by keeping his platoon alive by giving them jam fritters! Wonderful stuff.

~ ~ ~ ~ ~

Travelling by aircraft seems a daunting experience for anyone disabled, whether using a wheelchair or not, but in reality it isn't. It can be a seamless experience as you are helped every step of the way (that's not meant as a pun).

During my 26 years working for British Airways, I travelled to many parts of the world.

In fact in 1988 I travelled twice around the world, some 48,000 miles, in 5 days on aircraft, sponsored for charity. Not something I would recommend but the fact that I did it (as a full-time wheelchair user) shows you it's possible.

Stick to these guidelines and you will really enjoy the experience.

First, on booking your flight tell them you would like assistance from check-in to the gate. This could be a wheelchair with someone pushing or a lift on a golf type buggy. The gate could be over a mile away so don't think you're doing anyone any favours by not asking for help. The aircraft has a certain slot for take off; if you are late because of walking difficulties, THE AIRCRAFT HAS TO GO without you. Delays cost the airlines mega bucks.

If you have problems walking down the aisle when you get aircraft side, no problem: most aircraft now have small wheelchairs especially to take people up and down the aisle. If you can't walk whatsoever, no problem: tell them and facilities will be put in place from check-in to take you to the aircraft by ambulance, high lift you to the aircraft and trained medical staff will lift you into your seat. The golden rule here is: 'tell them'.

With some airlines you can pre-book your seat. If so, get one that has more leg room and is near the toilets, probably a bulkhead seat. The Civil Aviation Authority has made a ruling that no disabled person can have a seat by an Emergency Exit for obvious reasons.

If for some reason you get to your destination and your wheelchair is missing or worse still damaged, it is the airline's responsibility (assuming you're flying with a decent airline) under the Haig Protocol to restore or repair your chair. See the airline's staff and they will sort it out.

Things do go wrong and being calm, polite and firm is usually the best way to sort things out.

I remember I went to San Diego from Gatwick once and they left my chair behind. I was in a rush – had to get down to Tijuana – and the only one they had to loan me had a large sign above my head saying 'AVIS Rent a Car'.

The times I was stopped in my hotel by people saying, "Hey fella, where can I get a car?"

Flying's easy believe me, but it can hurt your arms!

---

***About the author***
*George Goodger was a bit of a tearaway in his youth, and hasn't really changed much.*
*Diagnosed with multiple sclerosis in 1973, he has been a full-time wheelchair user for 25 years, and is grateful that his condition has not deteriorated further since starting a controversial snake venom treatment in the 1980s and low dose naltrexone therapy (www.ldnresearchtrust.org) more recently..*
*George is now retired and dedicating his time to the development of © SillSave, a novel product designed to protect the sills and doors when wheelchair users transfer into motor vehicles.*

# About MS

Multiple sclerosis (MS) is the most common disabling neurological condition affecting young adults. It is the result of damage to myelin, a protective sheath surrounding nerve fibres of the Central Nervous System.

The symptoms in MS vary massively and any two people with MS will generally experience very different symptoms, many of which are invisible to others.

MS is commonly diagnosed between the ages of 20 and 40 and is incurable at the moment. For some it involves periods of relapse and remission, while for others it takes on a more progressive pattern.

# About the MS Society

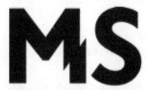

**Multiple Sclerosis Society**

Charity no. 207495

The MS Society is the UK's largest charity for people affected by multiple sclerosis (MS). It is a membership organisation but provide services to all.

The Society funds research, runs respite care centres, provides grants (financial assistance), education and training on MS. It produces numerous publications on MS, its symptoms and effect on daily life and runs a freephone specialist Helpline.

The MS Society is committed to bringing high standards of health and social care within reach of everyone affected by MS and to encourage and support medical and applied research into its cause and control.

The Society has a National Centre in London and offices in Northern Ireland, Scotland and Wales, along with a network of regions and branches across the UK.

## Governed by People affected by MS

As a membership organisation, the MS Society involves the MS community in all its activities and offers benefits for members, including the MS Matters magazine.

The MS Society board of trustees is elected from, and by, members of the MS Society. Every member has a right to vote in the elections and at the Society's annual general meeting.

## Our Aims & Declaration

As a charity, the MS Society aims to support and relieve people affected by MS and to encourage them to attain their full potential.

## Our fact file

The Multiple Sclerosis Society was founded in 1953 and is governed by a voluntary Board of Trustees.

For more information, please look at the MS Society website, www.mssociety.org.uk

# About the MS Trust

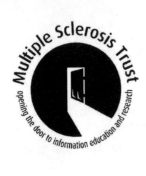

Charity no. 1088353

The MS Trust believes that everyone with MS should be able to live their lives to the full, and that everyone with MS should have access to an MS specialist nurse.

A national charity, we provide a free individual evidence-based information and enquiry service including a quarterly magazine "Open door", books and DVDs about dealing with MS. Our website is a huge resource of information, news and research about MS. You can contact us with any questions, write to us, email or call us and we will respond quickly to any request.

We are the specialists in MS education for nurses and therapists, including residential training courses for MS specialist nurses, and other education courses to reach as many nurses and therapists who work with people with MS as possible.

We make research grants for studies to help people with MS live their lives to the full. Recent research we've funded ranges from improving support to keep people with MS in work to a pilot study about the health benefits of vibration therapy, using a VibroGym system.

Finally, we are a campaigning organisation, working hard to increase the number of MS specialist nurses across the country and to drive improvements in MS services nationally.

We welcome all contact from anyone affected by MS, including friends, families, and the people who work with them.

For more information, please look at the MS Trust website, www.mstrust.org.uk or contact us at MS Trust, Spirella Building, Bridge Road, Letchworth SG6 4ET. Telephone 01462 476700 or email info@mstrust.org.uk

# About the MSRC

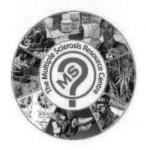

Charity no. 1033731

We are a national charity based in Essex and open to visitors or callers from 9 a.m. to 5 p.m. Monday to Friday. We also run the only 24 hour MS counselling line in the UK, manned by trained volunteers who either have or are affected by MS.

Our widely acclaimed glossy magazine, New Pathways, goes out to thousands of subscribers in the UK and abroad and the Editor, Judy Graham, is a renowned author on MS and related subjects.

The MSRC website has over 3000 pages of information, advice and much more besides and is easy to navigate and explore. Your personal MS stories, suggestions for links and items of general interest are all welcomed.

Our message board is a lively, inspiring and supportive place to visit and you can become as involved as you wish, whilst remaining completely anonymous if you prefer.

We understand that everyone with MS is a unique individual and we will treat them as such. We will always endeavour to help and advise people in such a way that they are capable of making their own decisions appropriate to their lives.

For more information, please look at the MSRC website, www.msrc.co.uk or contact us at Multiple Sclerosis Resource Centre, 7 Peartree Business Centre, Peartree Road, Stanway, Colchester, Essex CO3 0JN. Freephone: 0800 783 0518 Office: 01206 505444 or email info@msrc.co.uk

# About the Kent MS Therapy Centre

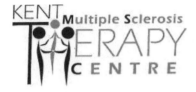

Charity no. 801382

The Centre was opened in 1984 with funds raised by a group of local people with MS who recognised the need for this type of facility.

Initially, the main aim was to provide hyperbaric oxygen therapy or HBOT (now more commonly known as high density oxygen therapy or HDOT). This involves breathing pure oxygen under pressure which many people with MS find improves certain symptoms such as chronic fatigue, bladder problems, pain and poor balance.

Oxygen therapy can also be used to treat many other conditions including cerebral palsy, stroke, leg ulcers, sports injuries and many more.

The Centre has evolved enormously since it was first opened and, like many other Centres around the country, now provides physiotherapy, reflexology, massage, counselling, chiropody, dietary consultations and clinics and workshops with MS Nurse Specialists and Continence Advisers.

Many people enjoy the benefits of the social aspect of the Centre, which provides an opportunity to chat to other people with MS in a happy, friendly and relaxed environment.

The present Centre has served East Kent well over the past 23 years but is now far too small for local needs. Patrons of the Centre are currently raising funds to build a new purpose built Centre to accommodate an extended range of services for those wishing to use them.

Friendly, professional advice is always available at the Kent MS Therapy Centre.

Merton Lane
Canterbury
Kent
CT4 7BA

Tel: 01227 470876 Fax: 01227 787395

Opening hours (2007):

9.30 - 1.30 Tuesday, Wednesday and Thursday


For more information, please look at the Kent MS Therapy Centre website www.kentmstc.co.uk


The Kent MS Therapy Centre is one of a nationwide network of independent therapy centres providing services to people with MS.

For your nearest centre, please look at the national therapy centres' website, www.ms-selfhelp.org